A Race Against Time

The Challenge of Cardiovascular Disease in Developing Economies

This report derives from a project conducted at Columbia University during 2003, which examined the economic and social consequences of cardiovascular disease in developing economies. The project followed on from the work of the Commission on Macroeconomics and Health, chaired by Professor Jeffrey Sachs.

ISBN 0-9754336-0-1

The principal investigators on the project were **Stephen Leeder, Susan Raymond** and **Henry Greenberg. Hui Liu** was a research associate. **Kathy Esson** served as a research associate and as contributing editor.

Stephen Leeder, MB, PhD, is Professor of Public Health and recently dean of the Faculty of Medicine at the University of Sydney. He is on study leave at Columbia University. He is a public health physician with a longstanding research interest in cardiac and respiratory diseases and the development of policies for their control. He has had extensive experience with health policy development with Australian federal and state governments.

Susan Raymond, PhD, is a global health and economic development consultant. She has been a senior advisor to the U.S. Agency for International Development and was Director of Strategic Planning for the New York Academy of Sciences. She has published widely on the changing economic and health care conditions of middle-income countries. She is currently a consultant to the Center for Global Health and Economic Development at the Earth Institute, Columbia University

Henry Greenberg, MD, is Associate Director of Cardiology, St. Luke's Roosevelt Hospital and Associate Professor of Clinical Medicine at Columbia University College of Physicians and Surgeons. He has a longstanding interest in international aspects of cardiovascular health, especially in the Russian Federation. He is currently a consultant to the Center for Global Health and Economic Development at the Earth Institute, Columbia University.

Hui Liu, MB, MS, MPH, is a graduate of Shandong University (China) and was a resident in medical oncology with the Chinese Academy of Medical Science/Peking Union Medical College. In the U.S., she obtained a Master of Science in Microbiology and Molecular Genetics from Rutgers University, and recently, her Master of Public Health from Columbia University.

Kathy Esson, PhD, is a social science researcher with special interests in public policy relating to education and health, equity and women's development and welfare. She has also worked as a psychologist and public servant in Australian federal health bureaucracies, health promotion programs and public inquiries. Her most recent project was as a senior member of a team conducting an independent inquiry into public education in schools in New South Wales, Australia.

Forewords

The Report of the World Health Organization (WHO) Commission on Macroeconomics and Health (CMH) in 2001 called attention to the two-way causation between health and economic development. Investments in health not only reduce the burden of disease, but also stimulate economic growth, which in turn raises a society's ability to invest in public health. On the other hand, when an economy is too impoverished to invest in health, it is likely to experience a devastating downward spiral of rising disease burden and deepening poverty. The CMH focused much of its attention on the urgent public health crises of sub-Saharan Africa, a region ravaged by HIV, malaria and tuberculosis. It did note, however, that cardiovascular deaths were set to increase from 3 million in 1998 to almost 5 million in 2020 in the WHO Demographically Developing Regions (without interventions), a year in which the number of deaths from infectious diseases and related conditions would equal the number of deaths due to chronic diseases. A central message of the CMH Report was that scaling up the investment in health, both from the resources available within a country, and with foreign aid when needed, was vital to enable the world's poorest places to escape from the trap of extreme poverty.

Following the work of the CMH, energetic efforts by the WHO with technical support from Columbia University have led to the formation of national macroeconomics and health commissions within many countries. These commissions examine ways to mutually enhance public health investment and economic development, based on the active cooperation of ministries of health and finance. Several of these national commissions have stressed that health concerns of macroeconomic consequence are not limited to infectious diseases, nutrition, and maternal health (the main areas of concern that formed the CMH agenda). Indeed, in many middle-income countries, physical injury and the non-communicable serious and chronic illnesses are of great significance. Not only do they translate into direct health care and social security costs, but they also reduce economic productivity by removing people from the active workforce. The following report on cardiovascular disease estimates that more than 6 million years of potentially productive life are lost in China each year because of heart disease and stroke. Thus, countries experience the economic impact of these cardiovascular disorders far beyond the health portfolio, including in industry and commerce, in households and in communities.

The report, sponsored by the Australian Health Policy Institute at the University of Sydney, the Earth Institute and Mailman School of Public Health at Columbia University, and the Initiative for Cardiovascular Health Research in the Developing Countries, seeks to integrate cardiovascular disease into the health-and-development framework adopted by the Commission on Macroeconomics and Health. This pioneering report is a first glimpse at the topic, using health and economic information, and the authors correctly stress the limits imposed by the available data. We now need more work to relate the impact of cardiovascular disease to the costs of interventions on a country-by-country basis. Likewise, large-scale attention to agricultural and food policy, tobacco control and city planning, all activities that could reduce heart disease and stroke, will need to be explored for their economic and political costs and benefits by each country.

This report paints a clear and strong argument, albeit in broad-brush strokes, that we need now to increase the attention we give to cardiovascular disease in low- and middle-income countries because of the combined health and economic impacts. This argument becomes even stronger in light of the emerging demographic profile of the world, where virtually every nation is now facing a change in the age structure of its population. The globalization of health-related knowledge and technology, although patchy, has been spectacular, and we are now enjoying the fruits of our success as life expectancies grow following decreased infant and child mortality. The time to act to minimize the impact of chronic disease is now, both to protect today's workforces and to diminish the burden of costly disability in the future.

I am very pleased that the team headed by Stephen Leeder has written this report, and I am most delighted that the Earth Institute has been able to support the project.

I commend the report to all those with an interest in health and development, and I expect that on the basis of this pioneering work, researchers and policy makers in public health and development will make important progress towards improved interventions regarding cardiovascular disease in many places in the world.

Jeffrey D. Sachs
Director, The Earth Institute
Columbia University
New York

When the WHO published the initial Report of the Commission on Macroeconomics and Health (CMH), many in the public health community were concerned that the Commission had not highlighted cardiovascular disease (CVD) and many other chronic diseases of global significance. The CMH Report did stress the importance of tobacco control as a priority for low- and middle-income countries but did not discuss other looming risks to the health of people in developing countries – like unhealthy diets and a lack of physical activity. This report by Stephen Leeder, Susan Raymond, Henry Greenberg, and their colleagues will start to dispel many myths that hamper progress in CVD and other chronic diseases. It will do so at a time when health has attracted the highest possible level of political interest globally – but for a rather narrowly selected number of infectious diseases.

Among the myths often cited and used as a rationale for inaction are that chronic diseases are mainly diseases of affluence affecting older people; that risks like smoking, unhealthy diets and a lack of physical activity are freely acquired and therefore government action is not warranted; and that infectious diseases should be controlled before addressing chronic diseases.

Leeder et al. emphasize the epidemiological and economic impact of CVD now and in the future. CVD will affect people in developing countries at younger ages than in developed countries; cause higher age-specific death and disability rates among them than those reported from developed countries when they experienced the peak of their CVD epidemics; and increasingly impact on poor people. Ischemic heart disease alone is anticipated to increase by 120% for women and 137% for men in developing countries between 1990 and 2020, compared to age-related increases of between 30% and 60% in developed countries. And the authors point out that this does not take account of increases in the prevalence of risks over time. Already information from over 100 countries shows that more 13 to 15 year olds smoke then ever before, and studies show that obesity levels in children are increasing markedly in countries as diverse as Brazil, China, India, and almost all small island states.

The economic and social dimensions of CVD are described in stark terms. For example, of the expected 9 million CVD deaths in China in 2030, over half will occur in the prime working ages 35-64. Figures are not much different for the other countries highlighted, namely, South Africa, Brazil, India and Russia. Overall, the authors state, "The proportion of CVD deaths occurring in prime labor years will greatly exceed the experience of U.S. and Portugal". And along with higher mortality goes higher morbidity and lower productivity.

While there is now a firmer basis to advocate for action, in my opinion the reality on the ground remains bleak for chronic disease control. As far back as 1956 at the Ninth World Health Assembly, a Resolution was proposed by India requesting the Director-General to set up an expert committee on CVD and hypertension. Almost 50 years later the capacity of countries to prevent and treat chronic diseases remains extremely weak. A recent assessment by the WHO[1] of 185 Member States provided information on various aspects of capacity. Most countries do not have budget lines for chronic diseases and report that essential chronic diseases medicines are not available in their primary health care clinics. The ability to develop integrated approaches to chronic disease prevention, surveillance and control remains rudimentary despite awareness of the need to act. Only a few developing countries, such as Brazil, Iran, South Africa and Thailand, have committed significant resources to chronic disease control. Developing countries often take their lead from donor and development agencies' priorities which to date have been largely neglectful of chronic diseases.

The intervention strategies outlined by Leeder et al. to address CVDs will contribute substantially to reducing the impact of other chronic diseases that share common risk factors with CVD. Thus many cancers, diabetes and chronic respiratory diseases could be prevented by stronger action against tobacco, unhealthy diets and physical inactivity. The rapid and full implementation of the Framework Convention on Tobacco Control and development of its protocols needs support that is more decisive. As well, significant financial and political support for the implementation of the WHO's new Global Strategy on Diet, Physical Activity and Health, has the potential to assist greatly in the control of three of the major risk factors driving the CVD and other chronic disease epidemics.

---

[1] Alwan, A., MacLean, D., and Mandil, A. Assessment of National Capacity for Noncommunicable Disease Prevention and Control. Geneva: the WHO; 2002

In addition, several academics as well as Leeder and his team have highlighted the potential for secondary prevention of CVD and diabetes in developing countries to prevent end organ damage and save lives in the short-term. We now need large-scale demonstration projects of impact to show the effectiveness of such approaches. The establishment of a health system that makes much use of primary care facilities to cope with both communicable and chronic diseases would improve overall population health. The new financing opportunities for chronic infectious diseases like HIV/AIDS and TB create a chance to build such integrated systems in the poorest countries.

At last, the public health community has a report that could stimulate debate and lead to action that will address CVD in much the same way in which Jeffrey Sach's original Report has helped to turn the tide on HIV/AIDS, malaria and TB.

Derek Yach
Representative of the Director-General
World Health Organization
Geneva

The last decade of the twentieth century greatly enhanced our awareness of the hitherto unrecognized global dimensions of the cardiovascular disease (CVD) epidemic. The Global Burden of Disease Study made it clear that accompanying the gratifying gains in cardiovascular health that occurred in the industrially developed nations towards the end of that century was an alarming escalation of the CVD epidemic in other and more populous regions of the world.

While the turbulence of political and economic transition unleashed an upswing in former socialist states, a post-colonial spurt in catch-up growth marked the health transition in the developing countries. While recent urbanization and delayed industrialization brought about sharp demographic and lifestyle shifts, globalization, the tail wind of the twentieth century, propelled the developing countries into the vortex of the global CVD epidemic. Events are now writing the history of these nations on the hearts of their people.

The first decade of the twenty first century offers us an opportunity to initiate action to counter these growing epidemics. The knowledge that is required to provide a comprehensive public health response is, for the most part, readily available. We need the effective application of that knowledge, through interventions aimed at populations as well as individuals, to reduce the risk of CVD across the lifespan in all regions of the world. Never before in the course of the cardiovascular epidemic have so many people been at risk of premature death, but also never before has such a vast body of knowledge been available which empowers us to reduce that risk. It is a challenge to human intellect and enterprise to apply that knowledge creatively and cost-effectively to minimize the future burdens of CVD in all regions of the globe.

A major barrier to the initiation of such action has been the lack of a compelling case, made to policy makers, that the CVD epidemics in low- and middle-income countries pose a serious threat to their development. The economic costs of neglected CVD epidemics were not apparent to influential opinion makers around the globe who assumed that CVD was principally a problem of the affluent and elderly in most nations. This study, on the macroeconomic effects of CVD in developing economies, helps to dispel that misconception by marshalling evidence on the adverse impact of mid-life deaths on economic and social development in those countries. The depletion of productive person power by CVD-related deaths and disabilities, which affect people in the labor force aged 35-64 years, should constitute a strong argument for initiating and implementing effective CVD prevention programs. The unaffordable demands that an unchecked rise in the numbers of people requiring high cost, technology-intensive, clinical care would place on health systems would also make CVD prevention the prudent choice.

Continued neglect of the CVD epidemic would mean that the poor among nations and the poor within nations would be the most vulnerable victims in the twenty first century. The low- and middle-income countries currently contribute about 80% of global CVD-related deaths and 87% of CVD-related disabilities. As the CVD epidemic matures, social gradients are reversing and the poor are becoming the major victims in all societies. The equity argument, too, works in favor of increased allocation of resources for CVD prevention and control.

The report also profiles pathways of action for cost-effective interventions that can provide a comprehensive response to the CVD epidemic in developing economies. These include macroeconomic interventions involving governmental policies, population-based health promotion and provider-based secondary prevention in individuals at high risk of CVD events. Recommended research pathways include in-depth country studies in four or more countries, to provide comprehensive economic analyses of CVD in their countries and to develop preventive strategies, as well as comprehensive community-based intervention trials to reduce hypertension and cardiovascular risk in at least three countries.

The Initiative for Cardiovascular Health Research in The Developing Countries (IC Health) is proud to be associated with this landmark study, as a sponsor and collaborator. IC Health will also be supporting the in-depth country studies that will follow and is developing projects for community-based intervention trials for CVD risk reduction in low resource settings. This report should help to break down the barriers of apathy towards the accelerating global epidemic of CVD and initiate much awaited but long delayed action for countering the threat it poses to developing economies.

K. Srinath Reddy
Professor of Cardiology
All India Institute for Medical Sciences, and Coordinator
The Initiative for Cardiovascular Health Research in The Developing Countries

Contents

Definitions and abbreviations used in this report

Definitions

More-developed countries: The richer, industrialized countries of the world; basically, the countries of North America, Europe, Japan, Australia, New Zealand, and countries of the former Soviet Union.

Less-developed countries: There is no fixed definition for these countries. They comprise the less rich and less industrialized countries of the world, but not those conforming to the definition of least-developed countries. They have already reached UN health and fertility goals or they will do so by 2050.

Least-developed countries: Countries designated by the UN using criteria of low per capita GDP, weak human resources (life expectancy, calorie intake, etc.), and a low level of economic diversification (share of manufacturing and other measures).

Middle-income countries: Countries having an annual gross national product (GNP) per capita equivalent to more than $760 but less than $9,360 in 1998. The standard of living is higher than in low-income countries, and people have access to more goods and services, but many people still cannot meet their basic needs for food and shelter. In 2003, the cutoff gross national income (GNI) for middle-income countries was adjusted to more than $745, but less than $9,206. At that time, there were about 65 middle-income countries with populations of one million or more. Their combined population was approximately 2.7 billion.

Low-income countries: Countries having an annual (GNI) per capita of equivalent to $760 or less in 1998. The standard of living is lower in these countries; there are few goods and services; and many people cannot meet their basic needs. In 2003, the cutoff for low-income countries was reduced to $745 or less. At that time, there were about 61 low-income countries with a combined population of about 2.5 billion people. All dollars are U.S. dollars.

Abbreviations

CGHED	Center for Global Health and Economic Development (Columbia University)
CHD	Coronary heart disease
CHF	Congestive heart failure
CMH	Commission on Macroeconomics and Health
CVD	Cardiovascular disease
DALY	Disability adjusted life-year
GDP	Gross domestic product
GNI	Gross national income
GNI PPP	Gross national income adjusted to purchasing power parity in U.S. dollars
GNP	Gross national product
HIV/AIDS	Human immunodeficiency virus/acquired immunodeficiency syndrome
IC HEALTH	Health Initiative for Cardiovascular Health Research in The Developing Countries
IHD	Ischemic heart disease
Mm Hg	Millimeters of mercury
mmol	Millimole chemical concentration
MONICA	Multinational Monitoring of Trends and Determinants in Cardiovascular Disease
MRFIT	Multiple Risk Factor Intervention Trial
NCD	Non-communicable disease
OECD	Organization for Economic Cooperation and Revelopment
PPYLL	Potentially productive years of life lost
UN	United Nations
UNESCO	United Nations Educational, Scientific and Cultural Organization
WHO	World Health Organization

A

Introduction

This report examines the social and economic impact of cardiovascular disease (CVD) in one low-income and four middle-income countries, now and for the next forty years. It also reviews strategies for the prevention of CVD in terms of their costs and benefits, where such data exist.

CVD is a major cause of morbidity and mortality in the world today and will become the leading cause of death and disability worldwide by 2020. (1) The diseases constituting its range of fatal expression (end organ CVD) include heart attack, myocardial infarction, acute coronary syndrome, congestive heart failure, strokes, kidney disease, and peripheral vascular disease.

The origins of CVD are located in society. High levels of CVD are found in environments where there is an abundance of food, where tobacco smoking is prevalent, where people do not take much exercise and where various strains and stresses operate. The dominant risk factors for CVD divide into modifiable and non-modifiable factors. Non-modifiable risk factors include age, gender, and genetic predisposition. The most important modifiable risks are tobacco smoking, high blood pressure, elevated blood lipids (hyperlipidaemia), obesity, and lack of exercise. The American Heart Association considers diabetes mellitus and its precursor condition – abnormal glucose metabolism due to insulin resistance, as seen especially in the metabolic syndrome discussed later – to be major risk factors for cardiac and vascular disease, as well as kidney disease. (2,3) Their increasing prevalence among children and adults in association with rising levels of obesity is of special concern.

These risk factors for CVD also constitute diseases in their own right; hypertension, hyperlipidemia, obesity and abnormal glucose metabolism are disorders that require medical intervention. These precursor conditions are major targets of CVD prevention in both populations and individuals. They accelerate the progression of pathological processes in vascular, cerebral and myocardial biology that over decades lead to end organ diseases such as stroke, heart attack and kidney failure, as well as the fatal arrhythmias that account for many of the sudden deaths that occur due to heart attack. These risk factors account for about 75% of coronary heart disease. (4) There is widespread agreement that risk factors are an appropriate focus of preventive efforts in relation to CVD in both developed and developing countries, because to the degree that an individual's risk factor profile is reduced, his or her susceptibility of developing end organ disease also decreases. The ability to treat these risk factors in individuals does not exclude interest in finding ways to counteract the forces in society that lead to high risk. These forces operate in the arenas of commerce, the economy and the environment. The impact of job strain, job demands and decision latitude has also been shown by Marmot and colleagues in the Whitehall studies of British civil servants to be additional determinants of CVD risk. (5) There is no reason to suppose that these risks are peculiar to one cultural context or one occupation.

The aging of all populations heightens the importance of CVD both in people of working age and in those who are beyond working age. Given the aging of the world's population from 1980 to 2040, we examine in detail the implications for selected developing countries. By 2020, the median age of the population in much of the developing world will begin to approach that of the West. In several developing countries this will create an age profile much like the West, but in so-called 'young' countries – those with a higher proportion of people aged less than 65 than found in, say, Europe – it will first produce a bulge of people of working age. The death and Δdisability attributable to CVD in labor force age groups in many of these countries may be much higher than that appreciated previously, and is certainly much higher than in Western nations now, and even in the past. Projections for the next two decades show that the mortality and disability rates attributable to these diseases will also rise.

The world has paid little attention to the chronic disease and disability profile of labor force, aged populations in the developing world. Even less has been paid to the economic implications of failing to stem current trends in the development and expression of these diseases.

In many countries undergoing rapid urbanization, the next twenty years will be ones in which the effects of rising CVD risk factors do their damage. Yet, because of the demographics of these countries, these years may not see the highest disease expression of these risks. CVD develops over several decades and is most prevalent in people as they grow older, and most of these countries are only slowly accumulating a significant number of older working people, or older retired people. In addition, the dependency rate (the number of dependants per working adult) will be low over the next twenty years, due to a combination of falling birth rates and a relatively small number of dependent elderly citizens.

There is an urgent need to act to stem the tide of risk factors that lead to CVD, in order to prevent a massive increase in the number of people with end stage illness. In our estimation, in young countries, while the levels of CVD risk factors are high, a two-decade window of opportunity exists to reduce their progression to end organ disease. If successful, the future costs of death and disability due to CVD will not become an intolerable burden. We have called this interval 'a race against time' to emphasize the importance of taking action now to prevent catastrophic levels of CVD twenty to forty years hence.

Fortunately, demonstrably effective interventions are already available for individuals at high risk of CVD. These disease prevention and management strategies significantly slow the progress of risk factors and prevent or postpone expression of their most serious end organ consequences. In addition, affordable public health and other public policy measures can readily be applied at the level of the population to ameliorate CVD's effects. These measures have been used to good effect in curtailing CVD in countries such as the U.S., Australia, the U.K. and other European nations since the mid 1960s. (6,7,8,9)

We explore the significance of CVD from both an epidemiological and an economic perspective. In reconciling the epidemiological projections with their likely economic consequences, we address the macroeconomic question: what will be the likely cost of CVD if we do nothing about it? Because there are now effective strategies for preventing and treating CVD, health officials can take decisions about investment in these strategies by considering the costs and benefits of intervention versus the costs and savings of doing nothing. Assuming that these explorations favor investment in intervention, health officials can make microeconomic choices – such as drug therapy or public health measures or a combination of both – based on cost-effectiveness data. They can choose among alternate investment strategies and determine budgets. We do not provide a detailed costing of the microeconomic implications of specific interventions to reduce CVD in this study. However, we do examine the limited evidence available in relation to both the cost and feasibility of individual and population-based interventions and locate it within the context of national government macroeconomic decision-making. For a complete analysis, we would need a lot more data on costs, especially those that concern the impact of CVD on the workforce.

The document begins by reviewing the derivation of this project from the work of the World Health Organization (WHO) Commission on Macroeconomics and Health. It then assesses the global significance of CVD. Five developing countries provide a case study to view the prevalence of CVD in low- and middle-income countries. Next, the macroeconomic implications of CVD are examined. Possible strategies to reduce the impact of CVD are then explored. And finally, we offer an agenda for action.

A-1. Origins and rationale of this report

In December 2001, the WHO received the Report of its Commission on Macroeconomics and Health (CMH). (10) The Director-General of the WHO, Gro Harlem Brundtland, had established the Commission to produce a comprehensive analysis of the relation between health and economic development. Seven working parties performed this work, and the CMH published a principal Report with six supplementary volumes. Professor Jeffrey Sachs, a professor of economics and then director of the Center for International Development within the Kennedy School of Government at Harvard University, oversaw the work of the Commission as its chair. Over 500 people expert in health and economics contributed.

The Commission strongly linked health to a macroeconomic perspective, portraying both health and health care as critical elements in country development, sufficiently important to engage the close attention of those responsible for overseeing each country's macroeconomic agenda. This departs from a conventional view of health expenditure that sees it as a sunk cost, and then assigns decisions about health service spending to the ministry of health, which then makes microeconomic choices about how best to invest the allocation they have received.

Central to the purpose of the Report of the CMH is the question so often asked by governments – why should we invest in health? Competition for public money is intense, even when it is for indisputably humane purposes. If investments in health and health services are to be justified, then the likely yield from those investments should compare favorably with benefits that would follow from the commitment of these funds to other purposes, including education, urban development, public transport, trade and industry, and defense.

Investments in health not only reduce the burden of disease, but also stimulate economic growth, which in turn raises a society's ability to invest in public health. On the other hand, lack of investment in health, due to overall economic impoverishment, has devastating consequences. The CMH Report focused much of its attention on the urgent public health crises of sub-Saharan Africa, a region deeply wounded by HIV, malaria and tuberculosis. It argued that increasing investment in health, harnessing a country's own resources and drawing on foreign aid when required, is essential if the world's poorest nations are to break out of a never-ending cycle of poverty.

The CMH Report argued that to improve economic well-being, more countries would need to invest more in public health measures including immunization, and in primary health care. It also confronted the uncomfortable reality that the necessary investment to achieve health gains and subsequent economic improvement is beyond the capacity of many of the poorest nations. In these cases, donor nations who sense the humane, economic and strategic importance of helping these countries out of their poverty must match or exceed the national financial contributions. The Report thus called for a manifold increase in donor commitment.

Whatever the source of the increased investments in health and health care, their management necessitates the involvement of ministries of finance and development, and even presidential/prime ministerial commitment to better health. The Report called on all nations to consider establishing their own commissions on macroeconomics and health where ministers of health and finance and their bureaucratic counterparts can meet to establish agendas for health and development. Several countries (e.g. Rwanda, Thailand, Djibouti, Jordan and the Sudan) have done this, the better to pursue these purposes.

The WHO, supported by a grant from the Bill and Melinda Gates Foundation, accepted the responsibility for implementing the recommendations of the Report. A technical support team in the Center for Global Health and Economic Development at Columbia University works with the WHO Commission on Macroeconomics and Health Secretariat in Geneva. The Center for Global Health and Economic Development (CGHED) within Columbia University is a joint venture of the Mailman School of Public Health and the Earth Institute. The present report on the challenge of CVD is a logical sequel to the CMH Report. We have examined the impact of CVD on the health and economic well-being of developing countries using the same mindset that led to the original recommendations from the CMH.

We are at a strangely paradoxical historical moment with regard to global health. Old problems coexist with new ones, and solutions to yesterday's crises provide the vehicle for tomorrow's threats. For example, under-nutrition remains by far the greatest risk factor for premature mortality among the world's least-developed countries. (11)

Improved nutrition has played a major role in health gain and economic development in many low- and middle-income countries. Yet now, excess and unbalanced nutrition threatens the health and well-being of many millions of people, a surprising number of whom live in countries that are not affluent. To this must be added one of humanity's greatest follies – tobacco smoking. The prevalence of tobacco use, which is now declining in developed countries is increasing in many developing countries, bringing with it death and disease.

The major non-communicable diseases (NCDs) that account for the vast bulk of the worldwide burden of illness, including CVD, often have their origins in lifestyles and socioeconomic conditions. These conditions reflect both individual and macroeconomic choices, the latter made at high levels both inside government and beyond. We can make a strong case to extend the macroeconomic approach to include a consideration of these disorders, chief among which are diabetes, heart disease and stroke. These have a close connection with agricultural policy, food marketing, tobacco production and sale, urban planning, employment, and education. This is not to argue that individual choice is unimportant in relation to lifestyle, but to recognize that the social, educational and economic context in which individuals operate powerfully, shapes the degree to which they can exercise choice.

B

The global significance of cardiovascular disease

B-1. What are the global data?

CVD currently contributes 30.9% of global mortality and 10.3% of the global burden of disease. (12) There are about 200 million people worldwide with clinically expressed coronary heart disease, stroke and other occlusive vascular diseases, and diabetes. Heart disease and stroke kill nearly 17 million people worldwide each year, compared to a death rate from HIV/AIDS of 3 million. Eighty percent of CVD deaths occur in low- and middle-income countries. In developing countries, CVD represents three quarters of the mortality from non-communicable diseases, and already accounts for 10% of the developing world's burden of disability. CVD is the principal cause of death and of much morbidity in industrialized nations. (11,12,13)

While CVD is a global killer, since the mid 1960s, deaths from heart attack have declined by more than 50% in many industrialized countries including the U.S., Finland and Australia (6,8,15) and similar declines have occurred for stroke. (7) In 1980 heart disease was the leading cause of death in the U.S. in the age cohort 45-64 and malignancy was second. (16) Age-specific data from 2000 show that malignancy is now the leading cause of death from age 35 through 74, albeit with a reduction in numbers of cases by 7.4% compared with 1980. Heart disease, now in second place in this age group, has fallen by 26% since 1980, and is now only the major cause of death after age 75. For heart disease, the age-adjusted death rate has fallen by 67%. (17)

The positive effects of action against CVD are readily apparent in industrialized nations where government agencies, medical leadership, and civic organizations have increased public awareness concerning the major CVD risk factors. Campaigns focused on diet, smoking and exercise, together with treatment of hypertension and high cholesterol, and surgical interventions when needed, have combined to have a major effect on CVD, reducing its mortality overall, and pushing it back from middle age to old age as a cause of death. Decisions taken at high levels of economic and legislative decision-making in several countries have contributed to these positive effects on cardiovascular health. CVD in these countries is now concentrated among older people.

Studies of the causes of the decline in CVD mortality in the U.S. and in other nations where CVD deaths have fallen have generally agreed that reductions in risk factors associated with diet (especially reductions in animal fat), smoking and exercise patterns accounted for half of the fall. These countries have achieved the other half of the reduction in heart disease mortality through progress in medical and surgical care, especially recently. This includes invasive and noninvasive methods of treatment concentrated on those with clinically expressed disease, and new and highly effective medications with which to treat hypertension and cholesterol. (17) The great unknown now is the effect of rising levels of obesity in many countries where falling CVD mortality has been a feature of recent decades. Will these increases lead to a recrudescence of CVD among younger people? This is a plausible possibility.

In essence, the effect of falling CVD mortality rates in the U.S. and similar countries has been to move the burden of CVD and other chronic diseases up the age ladder, with the positive impact of prevention manifest mostly in younger adults in their economically productive years. The less advanced the disease, the greater the impact of prevention, with risk factor reduction in younger people bringing the best results. Hence the most appropriate markers of a successful CVD prevention program will be a reduction in mortality overall, a shift in the peak burden of disease to older individuals (in terms of both mortality and morbidity), and control of the risk factors that lead to heart disease.

While in the developed world, prevention and treatment have pushed clinically manifest CVD to older and older people, in the developing world the age of onset of end organ disease grows younger. (18) In countries such as those of the former USSR, heart disease deaths today are far more common than in the West, although there are encouraging trends in several countries. (19,20,21) In Latin America, the Caribbean and the Middle East Crescent, heart disease also contributes greatly to mortality. In the heavily populated countries of China and India that account for more than a third of the world's population, CVD dominates the death toll, with millions of deaths a year attributable to CVD in each country (12,18,22)

CVD and diabetes are major causes of morbidity and disability as well as mortality. Disability comes with complex tentacles. Levels of disability vary, but if a disabled person cannot work, or must curtail his or her work, or requires care from another person, then the costs to the person and to society are substantial. In developed countries, social security safety nets bear most of the burden. In developing countries, where institutional care options are often lacking, care most often comes from another adult family member who is withdrawn from the workforce, or from a child, often a girl kept home from school. Indices of disease impact suggest that disability is as great a social and economic burden as premature death, and that CVD accounts for at least a third of all disability occurring among those over the age of 60. (23)

The growing burden of CVD in low- and middle-income countries follows the success of earlier public health initiatives. As Reddy et al. point out, life expectancy in India increased from 41.2 years in the decade 1951 to 1961, to 61.4 years for the 1991-1996 period, thus expanding greatly the population at risk of mortality and morbidity from all chronic diseases, including CVD. (18)

In 1971, Omran introduced the concept of the global health transition from communicable to non-communicable diseases as major causes of death. (24) He described the evolution of dominant societal health problems from infectious diseases and acute illness in the young to the non-communicable and chronic diseases, including CVD that are common in older people. Fox documents a longer history of non-communicable disease prevalence in the U.S., dating back to the turn of the 20th century. He also notes a puzzling avoidance of the prevention of non-communicable diseases by health policy leaders. (25)

The epidemiology of the health transition, and the particular role of CVD (including diabetes mellitus) worldwide, has been documented by multiple organizations and institutions. Foremost among these are the Global Burden of Disease project sponsored by the World Bank, the Health Sectors Priority Review, also sponsored by the World Bank, and the MONICA project sponsored by the WHO. (26,21,27) The U.S. National Institute of Aging has supported several studies. Investigators from Canada, India, Australia, New Zealand, Mexico, and the U.S. have also made substantive contributions to the growing database. (8,9,22)

Yusuf et al. explored the contemporary status of the epidemiological transition from infectious to non-communicable disease dominance. (12,15) They drew attention to the explosion of non-communicable diseases as a cause of mortality and burden of disease in most of the world. (12) In 1998, non-communicable diseases were responsible for 59% of total global mortality and 43% of the global burden of disease. Importantly, 78% of NCD deaths were borne by low-and middle-income countries, as was 85% of the NCD burden of disease. For CVD, the percentages were nearly identical. Looking at non-communicable diseases overall, by the late 1990s, nearly 50% of deaths worldwide were due to CVD, diabetes, cancer, and chronic lung disease.

Things are set to get worse. Projections suggest that for ischemic heart disease, a subset of CVD, the mortality for all developing countries between 1990 and 2020 will increase by 120% for women and 137% for men. Predictions for the next two decades include a tripling of ischemic heart disease and stroke mortality in Latin America, the Middle East, and even sub-Saharan Africa, a rate of increase that exceeds that for any other region, except for Asian and Pacific Island countries. By contrast, the increase in CVD deaths in more-developed nations, largely attributable to an expansion of the population of older people at risk, will range between 30% and 60%. (12)

The level of international attention paid to CVD in low- and middle-income countries has not matched its significance. As well, the potential for effective treatment and prevention in these countries is not fully appreciated. This is in part because CVD has few of the features that attract international sympathy or support. CVD rarely kills children. Adults with CVD do not provide heart-rending photo opportunities. There is no identified causal microorganism to treat with antibiotics or against which to raise vaccines. Rather, CVD is commonly seen as an affliction of affluence occurring in late middle and old age, a regrettable but inevitable feature of growing old, sometimes associated with victim-blaming. This view persists despite the fact that millions of people, especially the poor, die from CVD in their forties and fifties, and the social gradient in CVD is such that it is the poor, not the rich, who are generally most at risk. In countries with emerging economies, the onset of CVD occurs among ever-younger people. (18)

Instead, the great contemporary communicable diseases – HIV/AIDS, but also tuberculosis and malaria – and the health problems of children and women in their reproductive years have captured virtually all the attention and money devoted to international health problems. While a substantial response to these problems has been indisputably necessary, there is every reason to hope that as global health improves and economic development increases, it can be less exclusive and extend to include major non-communicable diseases such as CVD.

Raymond has shown that the first two decades of the present century offer a window of opportunity for much of the developing world to both manage contemporary chronic diseases in general and CVD in particular, and to respond energetically to the challenge of risk reduction to avoid unparalleled demands of chronic diseases in those aged 60+ in twenty years time. (29)

During these twenty years, while birth rates are falling and the number of people aged 60+ has not yet risen to the expected one billion, there will be a period when CVD is causing its principal social problems among those of working age. With decreased infant mortality and no substantial increase in the number of older people with disability attributable to chronic disease, the temporal and fiscal opportunity to set in place preventive and supportive health care systems is substantial. This period must not, however, be viewed passively: it is an opportunity requiring action of the highest order.

C

CVD status and projections in five developing countries

C-1. Methods and demographic profiles

The following section illustrates the role of CVD in the death patterns of one low- and four middle-income countries, now and in the future. These countries are Russia (with specific reference to the semi-autonomous republic of Tatarstan); Brazil (with specific reference to Rio Grande do Sul); India (low-income); China; and South Africa. We chose these countries to reflect the spectrum of CVD in mainly lower-middle-income developing countries. Russia has one of the highest rates of CVD amongst these nations, while South Africa has one of the lowest. The literature suggests that Brazil, India and China are on the cusp of facing a significant CVD problem. (12,18,28) We chose countries with a social security system and statistical collections that include social security and workforce data, however limited. We have a personal connection with each study country and they supplied data to us (see Acknowledgements at the end of the report). We used these data to draw pictures of CVD and its impact now and over the next 40 years.

We have used Portugal and the U.S. as two industrialized, high-income comparator countries. Portugal has the lowest CVD death rates in the European Union, especially among those under 65. The U.S. has high quality health and economic data, and has had, for several decades, aggressive CVD management and prevention programs. The process by which the U.S. has driven down CVD rates provides a backdrop for the potential for future action on the part of the five study countries analyzed.

We obtained CVD mortality patterns for countries from the WHO World Mortality Statistics 2003. (30) To predict CVD patterns at the national level over the coming three to four decades, we used population projections (by age and sex) from the

World Bank Development Indicators, 2003. (31) We used the year 2000 as the base year. We calculated death rates for CVD by age and sex from these tables and applied them to data from the changing demographic profiles of the study countries. In some instances we compare these data with data supplied by Dr. Colin Mathers (see acknowledgement p. 89) that have been adjusted for under-reporting and misclassification. We intentionally and consistently erred on the side of being conservative in our estimates. First, with regard to mortality, we used only published data on registered deaths and accepted the data at face value for each cause of death, without attempting to reclassify deaths into CVD from the category of uncertain causes. Second, we used only current death rates in our projections, assuming that future CVD death rates would not rise. We took this conservative position because we know that the data are weak. The real state of affairs then would be at least as serious as our calculations portray.

After examining current and projected CVD mortality figures for these countries, and exploring specific topics such as women's CVD mortality, we provide CVD projections for Brazil based on three sets of assumptions: things getting worse (risk factors increasing); steady state (2000 rates apply); and things getting better (based on the implementation of risk control strategies).

Table 1 lists the current population, per capita GNI PPP (gross national income adjusted to purchasing power parity in U.S. dollars) and health expenditure as a proportion of GDP for the five study and two comparator countries.

INDICATORS	S. AFRICA	INDIA	BRAZIL	CHINA	RUSSIA	U.S.	PORTUGAL
Population (million)	43	1032	172	1272	145	285	10
Per capita GNI PPP	10,910	2,820	7,070	3,950	6,880	34,280	17,710
Health as % GDP	8.6	5.1	7.6	5.5	5.4	13.9	9.2

Table 1: Population, per capita GNI PPP and health expenditure for the five study and two comparator countries, 2001.

Source: 2003 World Development Indicators, World Bank (31) and World Health Organization Statistical Information System (WHOSIS) [health expenditure]. (30)

Table 1 indicates the range of wealth of the five study countries, from South Africa, which is the most affluent in per capita terms, to China and India, which are the least affluent. All study countries have significantly lower per capita GNI PPP than the U.S. and Portugal. The study countries vary in population size from moderate (South Africa) to very large (India, China).

In terms of health expenditure, on average, 52% originates in the private sector in developing countries, coming overwhelmingly from household payments. This figure exceeds 60% in China and 80% in India. In more than half of all developing countries, more than 40% of their health revenue comes from private payments, and in a third, it is over 50%. In only 16% of developing countries does private payment account for less than 25% of total health care payments. (36)

Projected changes in population distribution in the developing world due to aging are staggering.

Figure 1 below illustrates the increase in numbers of people aged 65 and over in more-, less- and least[1]-developed countries, between 1980 and 2040. All three groups of countries have experienced and will continue to experience a significant increase in the population aged 65 and over. This is especially dramatic for those countries defined as less- (but not least-) developed. This category, which includes the five study countries, will experience a doubling of the population aged 65+ by 2020 and a more than fourfold increase by 2040, to almost 900 million people. The number of people aged 65+ will increase more slowly in the more-developed and least-developed countries. By 2040, the total number of 65+ citizens in more developed countries will be only one third of the number in less-developed countries.

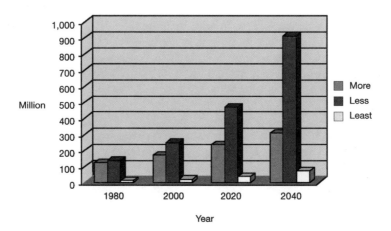

Figure 1: Projected increase in the population aged 65 and over from 1980 to 2040 in more-, less- and least-developed countries.

Source: United Nations Population Division. (32)

---

[1] Defined on page 3.

Figure 2 provides data on population increases for those aged between 35 and 64, the peak productive years. This figure indicates a leveling of the working age population in more-developed countries, but dramatic increases in least- and less-developed countries. While the numbers remain relatively small in least-developed countries, they increase dramatically in less-developed countries, to 5 billion in 2040. By 2040, the number of working aged people in less-developed countries will be more than five times the number in more-developed countries, and the number of working age people in least-developed countries will approach the number in more-developed countries.

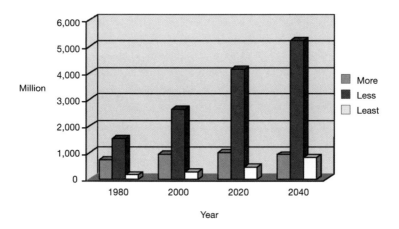

Figure 2: Projected change in the population aged 35-64 from 1980 to 2040 in more-, less- and least-developed countries.

Source: United Nations Population Division. (32)

Turning to the five study and two comparator countries, World Bank figures indicate that population changes will vary across the five study countries in the next forty years. India's population, on current indications, will increase to 1.5 billion by 2040, and will rival that of China. South Africa, Brazil and China will steadily increase in population, and Russia will decrease quite significantly.

Table 2 compares the current and projected population aged 35-64 and 65+ in the five study and two comparator countries for 2000, 2020 and 2040, expressed as percentages of the total population.

	S. AFRICA	INDIA	BRAZIL	CHINA	RUSSIA	U.S.	PORTUGAL
% population 35-64							
2000	25.8	27.0	29.5	33.2	40.0	38.5	37.0
2020	30.8	33.6	37.9	41.0	45.0	37.9	44.6
2040	34.2	38.3	38.0	37.4	38.0	35.0	37.2
% population 65+							
2000	4.7	5.0	5.1	7.0	12.0	12.7	15.0
2020	5.0	6.2	8.2	11.0	14.8	17.0	18.5
2040	7.9	10.2	13.9	19.7	20.0	22.4	26.8

Table 2: Current and projected population percentages for 2000, 2020 and 2040 for the five study and two comparator countries.

Source: 2003 World Development Indicators CD-ROM, World Bank. (31)

The patterns emerging here reflect those outlined for less-developed countries. Two trends stand out. First, while at present the proportion of people aged 35-64 is much lower in four of the study countries than in Russia or the two comparator countries, by 2040 the seven countries will have roughly equivalent percentages in this age group (between 34% and 38%). This represents a very significant increase in the working age population for the five study countries, especially for South Africa, India and Brazil.

Second, while all countries show an increase in the numbers of people aged 65 and over, there will still be differences among them in 2040 in the percentage of older people. South Africa, Brazil and India will remain 'young' countries, with only 8% to 14% of their population aged 65 and over. China and Russia will both approach 20% for this age group, and the U.S. and Portugal will be over 20%. Here, the distinction between the aging of the population and increases in the number of elderly people is important. Aging implies that the proportion of older people is increasing and that life expectancy is increasing, but in 'young' countries, this will manifest itself first in increased numbers of young adults and middle-aged people, more than in increased numbers of older people.

Both these trends reflect different effects of aging in the seven countries. Because CVD mortality increases as population longevity increases, this will have implications for all the study countries, in particular for China and Russia, and to a less extent for India, Brazil and South Africa.

Two implications of these trends are less well recognized, and they represent an opportunity and a challenge. First, across the five countries, as larger portions of the population enter the working ages, overall dependency rates will fall. The dependency rate refers to the number of people (the very young and the old, the numerator), who depend upon the workforce aged 15-64 for support (the denominator).

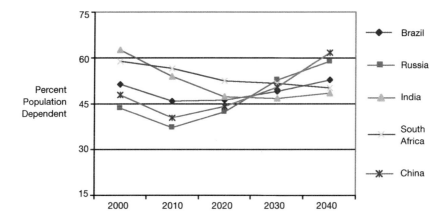

Figure 3: Percentage of population under 15 and 65+ (dependent) projected to 2040 in the five study countries.

Source: 2003 World Development Indicators CD-ROM, World Bank. (31)

Figure 3 shows that between 2000 and 2020 (and for countries like South Africa, beyond that), dependency will shift to below current levels for all five study countries. The demographic window of falling dependency represents a great opportunity for investment because the employed population will be supporting fewer dependants, and hence it is possible to allocate growth in incomes (personal, family and national) to investment.

Second, however, assuming present trends continue, the increase in the working age population in the five study countries will be accompanied by increasing levels of CVD risk factors and end organ disease in that age group. CVD mortality and morbidity is already high in this age group in those countries, and its rise will have serious implications for both health costs and productivity, not just in the next twenty years, but beyond. This could offset the benefit of a lower dependency rate. We explore the labor force implications of current and projected CVD rates later.

C-2. Overall CVD experience in the five study and two comparator countries

Table 3 presents a coarse-grained picture of CVD mortality in the study countries using crude death rates for CVD per 100,000 population as the summary statistic for CVD mortality in 2002. Because the figures were similar to those used by the WHO to calculate burden of illness, we quote their figures here.

INDICATORS	S. AFRICA	BRAZIL	CHINA	INDIA	RUSSIA	U.S.	PORTUGAL
Crude CVD death rate per 100,000 (2002)	199	225	230	266	945	317	391
Crude all-cause death rate per 100,000 (2002)	1481	695	105	985	1607	832	939

Table 3: Current crude CVD mortality and crude all-cause mortality in the five study and two comparator countries, 2002.

Source: C. Mathers (WHO).

However, as rates in industrialized countries decline, CVD death rates in middle-income countries are going up. A comparison of the age-standardized CVD death rates in the U.S. and the Russian republic of Tatarstan in **Figure 4** demonstrates this.

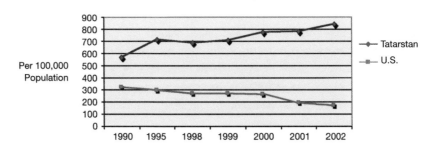

Figure 4: Age-standardized death rates per 100,000 population for cardiovascular disease in Tatarstan and the U.S. 1990-2000.

Source: (30) and Annual Health Statistics, 2002, Tatarstan Ministry of Health, July 2003; Kamil Sh. Zyatdinov, Minister for Health, Tatarstan and C. Mathers (WHO).

Figure 4 indicates that in the decade of the 1990s, U.S. age-adjusted CVD death rates declined by 20%, while rates in Tatarstan increased by 36%.

Projections of the number of deaths attributable to CVD in 2040 are even more deeply disturbing. We applied current age-specific mortality rates to the expected populations of the study countries for the next forty years.

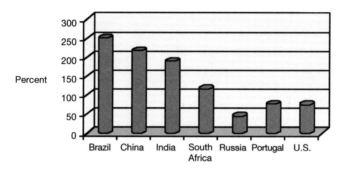

Figure 5: Percentage increase in the total number of CVD deaths for the year 2040 over the year 2000 for the five study and two comparator countries.

Source: Calculated from WHO Statistics Mortality Database (30) and 2003 World Development Indicators CD-ROM, WB. (31)

As **Figure 5** shows, even if we assume no increase in CVD risk factor prevalence, the total number of deaths due to CVD will rise tremendously in four of the five study countries relative to the U.S. and Portugal. This is because of their changing population structures. For this reason (the aging of all the world's populations), compared to 2000, the projected number of CVD deaths in 2040 in the population over 35 in four of our countries will be as much as two to four times higher than in 2000. Russia is the exception because demographers predict that its population structure will not change much over this period.

These figures translate into about nine million CVD deaths in China in 2030, over half of which will be in the prime working ages of 35-64. CVD is a growing problem in the five study countries whose actual importance will become clear only as their populations grow older.

C-3. Labor force implications

These disquieting figures of rising CVD burden in whole populations quickly pale, however, when we examine the patterns within CVD death rates relative to age groups. There, CVD in the five study countries is not a scourge of the aged. Rather it is a burden for the workforce right now, as we write.

C-3a. Mortality concentration in people of working age

Table 4 shows that in four of the five study countries (all except China), age-specific (35-64) male and female working age CVD death rates are significantly higher than in the U.S. or Portugal. In fact, within the working age populations of these countries, mortality rates from CVD are often equal to or greater than rates for the same age group in the U.S. before it embarked on the aggressive CVD prevention and management initiatives that have reduced its CVD mortality. Indeed, we have not seen the rates operating in Russia in the U.S. workforce for over half a century.

In India and South Africa, women's workforce death rates from CVD are also higher than those that U.S. women experienced in 1950. Men and women in Brazil aged 35-64 experience CVD mortality rates similar to those in the U.S. thirty years ago.

INDICATORS	S. AFRICA	BRAZIL	CHINA	INDIA	RUSSIA	U.S.	PORTUGAL
CVD death rate ages 35-64 (2000)							
Males	96.9	71	37.9	81	258.6	55.9	51.7
Females	68.2	48.9	23.8	55.9	63.7	27.9	17.9

Table 4: CVD age-specific mortality in the working age population in the five study and two comparator countries, 2000, expressed as a rate per 100,000 population.

Source: The WHO Mortality Statistics Database (30), WHO (for China and India) and UN Development Indicators CR-ROM (31).

For a problem so large, one would expect good quality data to be readily available, but they are not. The estimates in **Table 4** are low. We used reported deaths. We related the deaths to UN population estimates. Reported deaths are incomplete for many countries. South African data are about 50% complete, and for Brazil they are about 80% complete. The proportion of deaths coded to ill-defined causes varies across countries from a few percent in the USA to 10% in Russia, 20% in Brazil and Portugal and 40% in South Africa. (Colin Mathers WHO: personal communication). In South Africa Dr. Debbie Bradshaw and colleagues have adjusted data for under-registration and misclassification. This elevates the estimates in **Table 4** for males to 327 for men and 253 for women.

Figures from the WHO for men and women aged 35-59 are 187 and 156 (South Africa), 180 and 120 (Brazil), 91 and 62 (China), 211 and 139 (India), 576 and 179 (Russia), 116 and 53 (U.S.) and 99 and 35 (Portugal). Tatarstan may be a prime example of the future awaiting countries whose CVD death rates in their working age populations are even now cause for concern.

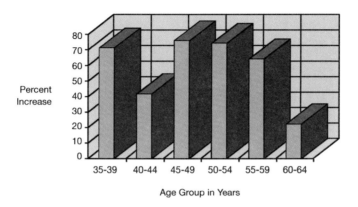

Figure 6: Percentage increase in age-specific CVD mortality rates in 2002 over 1984 in Tatarstan.

Source: Annual Health Statistics, 2002, Tatarstan Ministry of Health, July 2003; Kamil Sh. Zyatdinov, Minister for Health, Tatarstan

Figure 6 indicates that on average between 1984 and 2002, age-specific CVD mortality rates for those between 35 and 64 in Tatarstan increased by about 50%. Among men aged 35 to 39, the rate increase was an amazing 71% in less than 20 years. Currently in Tatarstan, the male CVD mortality rate is seven times the rate for this age group in Portugal and twice the CVD mortality rate among this age group 50 years ago in the U.S. Importantly, in Tatarstan, this trend in CVD mortality does not reflect a workforce that is getting sicker in general. Death rates for pulmonary disease, for example, among men between the ages of 35 and 49, have increased by just over 10%. Among men aged 50-64, pulmonary disease death rates have declined.

These numbers highlight what may happen in relation to CVD in less-developed countries. The technical capacity of their workforces will grow as less-developed economies grow. Members of these workforces require investment in training, and their loss in midlife through death is expensive to employers.

Another way of examining working age CVD deaths is to look at the percentage of deaths attributable to CVD rather than to other causes. **Figure 7** illustrates this for three of the study countries and the two comparator countries for males and females.

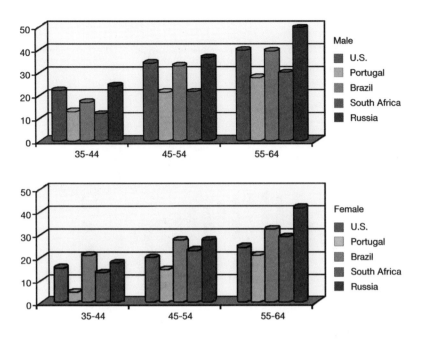

Figure 7: Percentage of male and female deaths attributable to CVD in 2000 by age group in the three of the five study countries and the two comparator countries.

Source: WHO Statistics Mortality Database (30)

For males, **Figure 7** indicates that the proportion of deaths attributable to CVD is approaching or has surpassed that for the U.S. and Portugal, especially so in Russia and to a lesser extent in Brazil. For females, the proportion of deaths from CVD is consistently higher in the three study countries than in the U.S. and Portugal, with women more disadvantaged relative to their counterparts in the U.S. and Portugal than are men.

The figures for Russia as a whole are consistent with the trends evident in Tatarstan, with just under 50% of male deaths and just over 50% of female deaths in those between 55 and 64 attributable to CVD.

CVD is already making inroads into the youngest workforce age group (35-44) that we studied. In Portugal CVD represents 12.9% of deaths in males and 5.9% of deaths in females aged 35-44. The comparable proportions in Brazil are 17.4% and 27.1%. HIV/AIDS in South Africa is both the principal cause of death at all ages (166,000 in

2000 and rising rapidly) and the cause of the most years of life lost (4,700,000 in 2000), but CVD of all forms accounted for 92,000 deaths in 2000. The proportions of deaths between 35 and 44 years attributable to CVD are 12% for men, and an amazing 17.2% for women. The South African picture is further illustrated in **Figure 8,** which shows that NCDs such as CVD make up an increasingly large proportion of causes of mortality as the population becomes older, and outstrip HIV/AIDS after age 45 in both males and females.

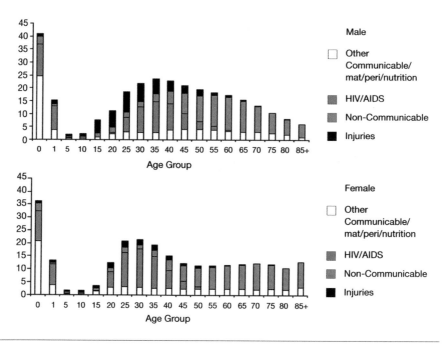

Figure 8: Thousands of deaths due to HIV, other communicable diseases, NCDs and injuries in South African males and females, 2000.

Source: Initial burden of disease estimates for South Africa, 2000. (33)

Figure 9 provides yet another illustration of CVD mortality rates in the study countries. It presents the percentage differences in male and female age-specific death rates in four of the study countries when compared with those in Portugal and the U.S. in 1999/2000. Thus in the top (Brazil), male death rates at age 35-44 are 40% higher than rates in Portugal and 30% higher than those in the U.S. For women, the comparable figures are 170% and 75%. In China (bottom panel of **Figure 9**), the CVD mortality is lower for men aged 35-44 than in the U.S. For women, higher death rates are seen in China for those aged 45-54 and 55-64 compared with similarly aged women in the U.S. and Portugal.

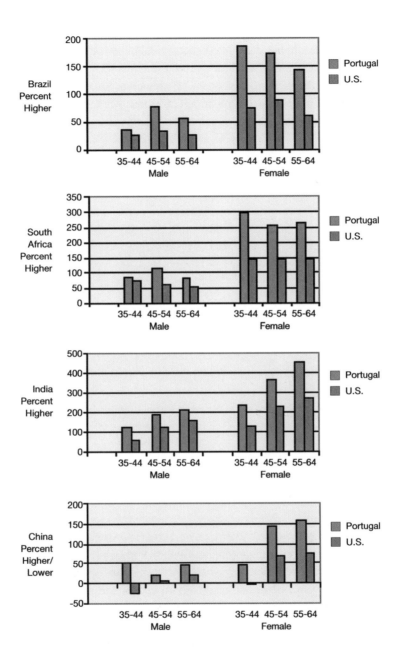

Figure 9: Using U.S. and Portugal CVD death rates as a base, comparisons of male and female age-specific death rates in India, China, Brazil and South Africa,1999 and 2000.

Source: WHO Statistics Mortality Database (30)

Although we do not present data beyond age 65, CVD deaths are concentrated in people of working age (35-64) in the four study countries to a degree not seen in industrialized nations. There is variation among countries, and presumably within countries such as India and China, but the sampled countries may not be extreme. The four countries have 30%-40% of their CVD deaths occurring in people of working age. The Philippines has over 50% of its CVD deaths in these ages, eight to ten times Western experience. This is attributable to two factors – first, these countries have higher age-specific mortality rates for those of working age and, second, they have larger populations of working age at risk and smaller older populations compared with the U.S. and Portugal.

In addition, while CVD occupies a variable position in the death patterns of working age men, in nearly all equivalent age groups CVD accounts for a greater portion of female deaths than in the U.S. or in Portugal. We address the consistent and striking importance of CVD for women's health in C-3d. below.

C-3b. Workforce CVD mortality projections to 2030

The picture becomes even grimmer when we project working age deaths from CVD in the study countries, using the WHO mortality rates and World Bank population projections. (29,30) In making these calculations, we assumed no increase in CVD risk factors over the 30 years and stable susceptibility to these factors so that the age-specific rates remained steady. We have already commented on the variability in death data, but this should be less of a problem here when we are comparing death rates in the same population at different ages and dealing with proportions of deaths. Increases in numbers of deaths at different ages in this calculation, therefore, are due to larger populations at risk. **Figure 10** illustrates cumulative CVD deaths from 2000 to 2030 for all countries disaggregated by age group.

For all countries, the greatest cumulative proportion of CVD deaths will occur in those aged 65 and over, ranging from 59% in South Africa to 91% in Portugal. However, what is perhaps most striking is the comparative cumulative CVD death percentage for those between 35 and 64.

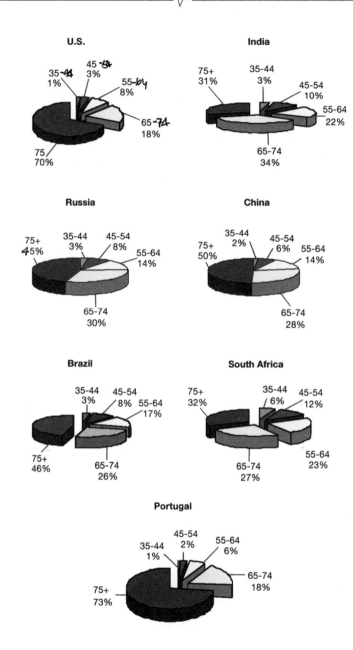

U.S.

35-44 1%
45-54 3%
55-64 8%
65-74 18%
75 70%

India

75+ 31%
35-44 3%
45-54 10%
55-64 22%
65-74 34%

Russia

75+ 45%
35-44 3%
45-54 8%
55-64 14%
65-74 30%

China

35-44 2%
75+ 50%
45-54 6%
55-64 14%
65-74 28%

Brazil

35-44 3%
45-54 8%
55-64 17%
75+ 46%
65-74 26%

South Africa

75+ 32%
35-44 6%
45-54 12%
55-64 23%
65-74 27%

Portugal

45-54 2%
35-44 1%
55-64 6%
65-74 18%
75+ 73%

Figure 10: CVD deaths distributed by age group for each country. Deaths are three-decade totals for CVD 2000-2030 in each age group.

Source: WHO Statistics Mortality Database 2003 (30): Tatarstan Ministry of Health, July 2003; Kamil Sh. Zyatdinov, Minister for Health, Tatarstan

Table 5 makes this explicit. It presents the percentage of CVD deaths for this age group for the study countries, the U.S. and Portugal accumulated across the years from 2000 to 2030, the same numbers used to produce **Figure 10.**

S. AFRICA	INDIA	BRAZIL	CHINA	RUSSIA	U.S.	PORTUGAL
41%	35%	28%	22%	25%	12%	9%

Table 5: Cumulative percentage of all CVD deaths, 2000-2030, occurring in males and females aged 35-64 in the five study and two comparator countries.

Based on these figures, all the study countries, but especially India and South Africa, are expecting a dramatic number of working age people to die of CVD over the next 30 years. In China 4.5 million CVD deaths will occur in 2030 in people aged 35-64. Because of a growing population of younger people at risk of CVD in the five study countries, the proportion of CVD deaths occurring in the prime labor years will greatly exceed the experience of U.S. and Portugal. This phenomenon is demonstrated by comparing Brazil's 35-44 age group in 2020 with a cohort of the same age in 2000 **(Figure 11)**.

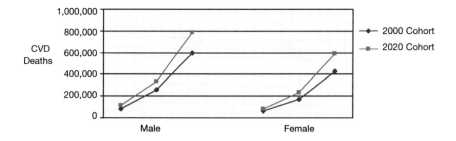

Figure 11: For 35-44 year olds in 2000 and 2020, a comparison of number of deaths attributable to CVD in each of three subsequent decades, assuming stable age-specific mortality rates and changing demographic structures.

Source: Calculated from WHO Statistics Mortality Database (30) and 2003 World Development Indicators CD-ROM, WB. (31)

CVD takes a lot of lives in both cohorts by age 64. Because demographic aging places more individuals in these age groups by 2020, we expect that the combined male and female 2020 cohort will experience a total of 2.1 million CVD deaths in 30 years, 33% more than the 2000 cohort will suffer.

Who is likely to be most at risk of early death and disability from CVD? If the experience in the West applies, elites in developing countries will be the first to realize the need for behavioral and other changes to reverse their risk. Those who are less educated and less wealthy – factory workers and semi-skilled suburban dwellers – will be more likely to keep smoking, eat high fat food and not act to protect their health. In addition, in several of the five study countries, these individuals will have less access to high quality, affordable health care than their more privileged compatriots do. The ongoing burden of CVD death and disability is likely, therefore, to fall on the poorer (although possibly not the very poorest) sections of society, as it continues to do in more- developed countries.

C-3c. Higher morbidity in working ages

Where we have morbidity data indicators (such as hospital admission data) for the five study countries, they are consistent with, and indeed perhaps more striking than, the death patterns. In Rio Grande do Sul, in Brazil, with the exception of stroke in ages 35-44, the hospital admission rate for working age men and women with heart disease and stroke is higher than the average hospital admission rate for this age group for all conditions **(Figure 12).** In other words, doctors admit working age men and women to hospital for CVD diagnoses at higher rates than for other illnesses.

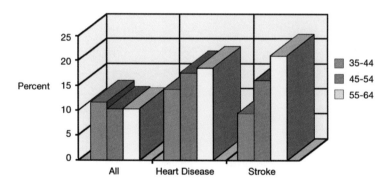

Figure 12: Percentage of admissions by age group for all causes in Rio Grande do Sul, Brazil, compared to age distribution of admissions for cardiovascular conditions and stroke.

Source: Brazil Ministry of Health; http://www.datasus.gov.br 2003

In addition, age-adjusted morbidity rates per 100,000 working age population in Rio Grande do Sul are four to five times the CVD working age mortality rates in Brazil, as shown in **Figure 13.** This indicates that there is a huge wave of illness among working age people. This in turn will contribute to higher working age death rates and hospital admissions and pulse forward into higher death rates after age 65.

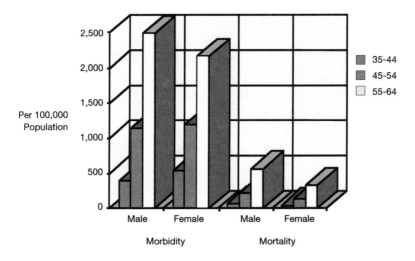

Figure 13: CVD morbidity rates in the province of Rio Grande do Sul and CVD mortality rates in Brazil overall.

Source: Brazil Ministry of Health; http://www.datasus.gov.br 2003

Admission to hospital is only one reflection of morbidity, and much hypertension and CVD goes undiagnosed and hence untreated, in or out of hospital. Surveys in Tanzania, for example, indicate that only 20% of people with elevated blood pressure in the surveyed populations were aware of their hypertension, and only 10% were receiving therapy. (34)

South African hospital data show a less striking pattern, but one that indicates that South Africa's CVD problem is likely to persist. We examined CVD hospital claims data from a private insurance company covering 14% of the insurance market in South Africa. We recognized that these data might over-represent the CVD problem in South Africa as a whole, because they cover only the more affluent formally employed population among whom medical care for CVD is more common. In this context we assumed, conservatively, that the 14% insurance coverage represents 20% of CVD hospital admissions in South Africa.

Claims data for hospital admissions by diagnosis indicate that for every CVD death in South Africa, there is one CVD-related hospital episode. Hence, hospital morbidity rates are about equal to mortality rates. Again, this underestimates the problem, because in South Africa which has a well-developed medical system, physicians handle much CVD morbidity in outpatient settings.

All of the data presented in this section on workforce implications of CVD rates in the five study countries indicate that the importance of aging for these countries is not (for now) the emergence of the aged, but (at present) the disproportional impact of CVD within the younger, most important economically productive years of life. In the five study countries in the next decades, demographic aging will exact its health and economic cost not so much among the older ranks as among workers.

C-3d. CVD and women's health

Health experts and the media rarely portray CVD as a women's global health problem. In developing nations, global health efforts have more frequently, and often exclu-sively, concentrated on women's maternal and reproductive functions. Examining working age data by gender, however, raises a caution about that focus and forces a reconsideration of its exclusivity. The impact of CVD on women is both direct, when they experience the illness themselves, and indirect, when their educational and economic circumstances are affected by death or disability due to CVD of family members.

For the five study countries, CVD can be as important, or more important, a cause of morbidity and mortality in women as it is in men, especially relative to population structure. For example, in Brazil, Russia, and South Africa, CVD in 2000 accounted for a higher proportion of all deaths for women than for men, although the total number of deaths was lower for women. Indeed, in South Africa in 2000, even with the over-whelming presence of HIV/AIDS as the leading cause of death, CVD ranked third in terms of women's disease burden, whereas it was sixth for men. Among South Africa's non-communicable diseases, the CVD burden comes to rest most heavily on poor women. In South Africa, CVD causes the highest portion of years of life lost due to NCDs for poor women: 45.5%, compared to 35% and 36% for poor and wealthy men respectively. (33) CVD may be equally consequential for women in other African countries. Although only focused on stroke, a study of urban and rural populations in Tanzania found that stroke death rates were proportionately higher for urban women than for urban men. (35)

Referring back to **Figure 9,** although women in the four study countries had lower CVD death rates than men, women in these countries overwhelmingly had higher death rates than comparable women in the U.S. and Portugal in 1999-2000. The differences are particularly striking in relation to Portugal. Moreover, the difference between women in the four countries and women in the U.S. and Portugal was always greater than differences among men in these countries and men in the U.S. and Portugal. This is true for all of the countries, as well as for the three countries in a study done for the Agency for International Development that included the Philippines, Thailand, and Mauritius. (36) It is not clear why this is so.

The differences between women in the five study countries and their counterparts in industrialized countries are also illuminating when measured not as overall death rates, but as the importance of CVD in the mortality patterns of younger women (see **Figure 7).** While CVD accounts for a smaller number of deaths among women than among younger men in the five countries, it constitutes a larger proportion of deaths for younger women compared to their U.S. and Portuguese counterparts. In South African women aged 35-44, for example, the proportion of deaths due to CVD is 17.4% compared to 5.9% in Portugal, and for women aged 45-54 in Brazil it is 36% compared to 26% in the U.S.

Women will continue to experience disproportionately high mortality from CVD. By 2040, women in the study countries will represent a higher portion of CVD deaths than their gender's portion of the population. In 2040 in China, for example, women are projected to be 49.5% of the population, but even if death rates no higher than now apply then, they will represent 54.6% of CVD deaths. In Brazil and China, the growth of CVD deaths among working aged women between 2000 and 2040 will be higher than for men. (30,31)

CVD morbidity can also disproportionately affect women. In Rio Grande do Sul, our investigations indicate that women have higher rates of CVD morbidity (as measured by hospital admission) at all age cohorts for working ages than do men. When con-genital heart disease is removed from these morbidity data, women still have overall higher morbidity rates than men, especially in the 35-44 age group.

It is also important to view CVD within the context of women's health in the child-bearing years and during the years of family formation and development that follow prime childbearing years. In the study countries, CVD appears to be on its way to playing a much more important part in those years than has been recognized to date. In all five countries studied, CVD accounts for a larger portion of overall female deaths than conditions related to childbearing, a point that often goes unrecognized due to the stereotype of CVD as a disease only of older women. (38)

In Brazil, the number of CVD deaths in women aged 15-34 is twice that from pregnancy-related causes. In addition, the number of Brazilian CVD deaths in the decade after prime childbearing years, 35-44 years, is nearly five times the deaths from pregnancy-related causes during the two decades of ages 15-34. This pattern also applies in China where there are 61% more CVD deaths in women aged 15-34 than deaths from maternal conditions. (30) In subsequent decades, three times as many women will die from CVD as died of maternal conditions in the previous two decades. (38)

In Russia, the differences are greater. CVD deaths among women aged 15-34 are four times pregnancy-related deaths. Female CVD deaths in the single decade after prime childbearing years are nearly 20 times all maternal deaths in the two decades of prime childbearing. There are clear implications here for definitions of health risk to women in developing countries.

Global health analysts should reconsider the current narrow definition of health risks to women in developing countries, and move beyond an exclusive concern with maternal and reproductive problems to include the profound impact of chronic diseases such as CVD. CVD should become a new priority for women's health.

C-3e. Widowhood

Workforce CVD deaths in men also cause havoc for married women by making them widows. Notwithstanding the death toll among women, the higher heart disease rates among young men in the prime of life mean that CVD is creating an equivalent cohort of widows who need support for decades. When 40-50% of men die before age 64, but only 25% of women die by age 64, the consequences are self-evident.

The study of widowhood and poverty is only beginning in the developing world. Data from the U.S. indicate, however, that the earlier women are widowed the more likely they are to live in poverty at older ages. In the U.S., nearly 35% of women widowed at age 55 whose widowhood lasts 6 to 10 years live in poverty, compared to 10% of women widowed at age 65. (37)

There are no comparable data for developing countries. Age-specific data are not universally available. U.S. Census Bureau data indicate that between 47% and 55% of women aged 60 and over in the five study countries are widowed. (38) Widowhood happens to many of these at young ages. In China, 20% of all widows are aged 35-59. (39) Surveys of Muslim widows in Delhi reveal that as many as two-thirds may become widows between the working ages of 30 and 60. (40) Examination of census data in Sri Lanka indicates that nearly a third of women aged 60-64 are widows. (41)

Some isolated studies indicate that one of the fastest paths to poverty in the developing world is widowhood. UN data show that in Brazil, the percentage of women widowed rose from 5% in 1970 to 8.1% in 1991. By 1991, 52% of the nation's widows were under the age of 65, and 16% of the women aged 45-54 were widows. The 1991 Brazil census found that 57% of women over 65 but only 17.5% of men over 65 were widows and that women were more likely to live in poverty than men were, in part because until recently, social security payments did not cover widows. (42) In India, only 15-20% of widows remarry. (43)

Urbanization will matter greatly in this relationship. In India, where employment rates in the years 35-64 for urban women are only 20%-30%, the loss of men of working age is devastating to household viability. In fact, in India, women's labor force participation rates in urban areas for all decades from age 35 to age 64 have declined since 1977. As urbanization grows, and CVD death grows apace, the loss of men will have heavy impacts on women. (38)

C-3f. What will happen if CVD risk factors get better or worse?

Sobering as it is, the increases in mortality attributable to CVD that we have projected for men and women in developing countries during their working years assume that nothing else gets worse. But, over time, the prevalence of many CVD risk factors is also likely to increase in these countries. In particular, higher levels of smoking, overweight, diabetes and high blood pressure will put people at even greater risk than they are at present. A range of factors contributes to this trend in developing countries, including the impact of industrialization, urbanization, globalization and increasing wealth.

Increased urbanization is associated with a growing labor force and an aging (although not necessarily old) population. One of the reasons why urbanization has been possible is the spectacular increase that has occurred in efficiency of agricultural production. This has had two major effects, the first being to release a substantial rural workforce that can now devote its labor to tasks in cities. Second, food consumption patterns are changing. Nutritionists estimate, for example, that the prevalence of under-nutrition in the developing world will fall from 17% now to 6% by 2030.

By then, food consumption will provide on average nearly 3000 kcal per capita per day. (44) Urbanization is also directly associated with economic growth. Indeed, in China, economic strategists are encouraging planners to accelerate urbanization, projecting that a 1% increase in urbanization annually will add 3% to economic growth. (45) Even in Africa, estimates are that half the population will be urban by 2020.

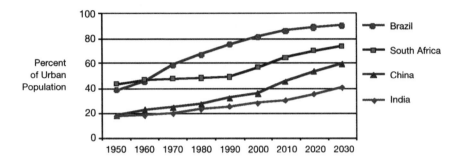

Figure 14: Percentage of population living in urban areas by decade 1950-2000 and projected to 2030.

Source: World Urbanization Prospects, UN, 2002 (49)

Figure 14 indicates that for four of the study countries, there will be a steady increase in the percentage of the population living in urban areas between 2000 and 2030, especially in Brazil and South Africa, but also in China and India (Russia is already urbanized). This reflects a trend that has been occurring for several decades. In Brazil, already predominantly urban, 90.5% of its population will be urban by 2030. Brazil's urbanization has occurred at all levels of city-size and throughout large sections of the country. (46) By 2030, 73.5% of the population in South Africa will be urban, 59.5% in China, and even 40.9% in India. (47) In India, there were five cities with over 1 million residents in 1951. By 2021, there will 51. (48)

The move to cities is an important factor influencing CVD and its risk factors. In India, risk factor profiles are far more intense in urban populations. Among a sample of 35-64 year old men, urban hypertension rates were two to three times those of rural areas. Data from the mid-1990s indicate that two-thirds of urban Indian men aged 35-44 have at least one risk factor for coronary disease. By age 45, the percentage is three quarters. While a bit more than a third of urban women age 35-44 have at least one CVD risk factor in India, by age 55 that portion has risen to 80%, being higher in the cities than in rural areas. Overall CVD prevalence in urban Delhi was 87.2 per 1000, compared to 44.8 per 1000 in rural areas surrounding Delhi. Currently, 28% of India's population is urban. If this rises to 40% by 2040, and the urban prevalence rate stays the same, this will result in more than a 75% increase in CVD cases in urban areas.[2]

In South Africa, CVD mortality rates in a survey of northeastern rural areas were 40% lower in those aged 55-74 years than South Africa's overall rates, indicating that urban rates must be much higher than rural rates since only 48% of the population is urban. (50) A 1998 survey in South Africa found that 26.4% of women were obese and that 36.6% of women known to be hypertensive had their illness controlled with medication. In general, awareness of hypertension and the use of medication increased with income. Hypertension was only half as common among rural as among urban women. (51)

Saturated fat intake, sodium intake (as measured by urinary sodium), and body mass index all appear to be rising in developing countries, with higher rates in urban areas than in rural. In many countries, urbanization is associated with steadily increasing rates of obesity, not least because that environment enables individuals to respond to market pressures to consume more food than they need and to exercise less than they need. (11) In Asia, a steep increase in stroke mortality has accompanied a rapid rise in the prevalence of hypertension. In surveys in India, The Philippines, Thailand, Sri Lanka, Pakistan and Nepal, hypertension prevalence (>140/90 mm mercury) varied between 15% and 35% of the urban population, with rural rates two to three times lower, a matter considered worthy of research by local experts interested in CVD control. (52,53)

In India, a rural and urban study as long ago as 1989 found values of body mass index, blood pressure, cholesterol, and diabetes in cities to be approaching those of Indian populations who now live in industrial countries; and there is no evidence that these trends have slowed down. Recent rates of increase indicate that in India, the proportion of people overweight (including those who are obese) will increase from 9% to 24% between 1995 and 2025. (54) Overweight is also set to rise in China. Projections for China, for example, indicate that by 2025, 37% of men and 40% of women will be overweight, compared to 8% and 12% in 1995. (55) Overweight is a risk factor for both hypertension and diabetes, with projections suggesting that in

---

[2] Data obtained from Rapp. *trimest. statist. sanit. mond.* 46 (1999) page 104: Table 4 Repartition des sujets en fonction du nombre de facteurs de risque coronariens modifiables dans un echantillon de la population urbaine, en Inde, and Table 5 Tendence et projections demographiques en Inde,1981 à 2021.

China, hypertension will increase from 18.6% to 25%, and diabetes from 1.4% to 2.4% between 1995 and 2025. In India, the equivalent figures are 16.3% to 19.4% for hypertension and from 2.1% to 3% for diabetes. (54)

According to the WHO, worldwide deaths attributable to cigarette smoking are expected to nearly double, from 5 million to 10 million a year, between 2000 and 2020. In India, projections estimate that tobacco-attributable mortality will grow from 1% in 1990 to 13% in 2020. In Brazil, studies of acute myocardial infarction indicate that heavy smoking is the most important risk factor for early heart attack. (56)

In developing countries, risk factors often increase with rising incomes (hypertension and obesity) in part attributable to a changing diet that has more fat, salt and calories, and to increasing body weight and less exercise among the affluent. But other risk factors tend to be more prevalent among lower income groups (both light and heavy smoking). These factors are generally more common in urban than in rural communities. Over time, experience in western countries suggests that the more affluent sections of society adjust their lifestyles in directions that favor heart health, with CVD risk then concentrated among the less advantaged. (8) These figures do not mean that CVD is not, and will not be, an increasing problem in rural areas. Cause of death data from rural India show that from 1992-1997, CVD increased from 8% to 12% of deaths. (30) Still, there are indications that CVD patterns for cities are higher than for rural areas. Although migration from rural to urban areas by sick people seeking care may explain part of the rural-urban gradient, it does not explain much of it. Most is due to changes in diet and physical exercise.

One can estimate broadly the impact of a combination of aging, a growing urban workforce, and rising CVD risk factors on CVD morbidity and mortality. In China, based on past trends and projected increases in risk factors, a 215% increase in CVD death rates seems likely in the 30-year period, 1995-2025. (55) To examine further the likely impact in the five study countries, we estimated future CVD mortality based on increased, decreased and steady state CVD risk factor prevalence. **Figure 15** illustrates these three future scenarios for Brazil. It shows starkly the imperative to act now to forestall future increases in CVD mortality.

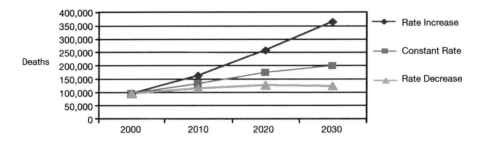

Figure 15: Brazil: annual CVD deaths in the 35-64 age group in 2000, 2010, 2020 and 2030, under conditions of constant 2000 CVD death rates, increased rates and decreased rates.

Source: WHO Statistics Mortality Database (30) and 2003 World Development Indicators, WB (31)

We assumed that due to increases in CVD risk factor prevalence, the 35-44 year old age group in Brazil would experience a 15% increase in CVD mortality rate per decade over 30 years. We based that assumption on the projected rates for China (see above) but to be conservative, thought that the increase in CVD death rates in Brazil would be less than the documented increase in Tatarstan and less than that projected for China. Similarly, we assumed that the 44-54 year old age group would experience a 20% increase, and the 55-64 age group a 25% increase.

First as a result, the labor force by 2030 will experience an 84% increase in CVD compared to the number of deaths, if the current death rate persists. The top line in **Figure 15** represents this scenario. While this figure falls well short of the projected CVD increases in either China or Tatarstan, the price of doing nothing about risk factors and management of early CVD is clearly high even in Brazil. Given the certainty of rising risk without prevention, CVD rates will increase, and without preventive disease management these rates will lead to new waves of excess morbidity and mortality.

Second, returning to the middle line of **Figure 15,** a steady rate of age-specific CVD mortality still sees an increase in number of deaths by 2030, due to demographic changes. Failure to hold cardiovascular risk factor and disease rates to even their current high levels will exact a tremendous price in developing countries, especially in the Brazilian workforce over the next three decades.

Third, action now to prevent both an increase in those with CVD risk factors and those with clinically expressed CVD will pay significant mortality dividends over 30 years.

The bottom line in **Figure 15** uses decadal declines in the U.S. CVD death rate, which for the 35-64 age groups, have varied from 10-15% in the 1950s to 25-35% in the 1980s. We might expect that these rates would apply to countries that instituted similar CVD control programs to those that were associated with these declines in the U.S.

If we assume that Brazil instituted control programs that achieved a decadal rate reduction of 15% of deaths among men aged 35-64, compared to constant rates, this would result in a 15% decline in the number of CVD deaths in the decade to 2010. This in turn would lead to a 28% decline in the number of deaths in the next decade to 2020 and a 39% decline to 2030. However, this does not imply a significant reduction in numbers of people dying. The denominator at risk will continue to increase due to demographic factors. Rather, it holds numbers of deaths relatively steady, as indicated by the third and lowest line in **Figure 15.**

D

The macroeconomic and economic consequences of CVD

The previous sections hint at the potential economic costs of CVD and its risk factors. In this section, we explore the costs of CVD more closely.

To develop an estimate of the macroeconomic consequences of CVD we have calculated the years of productive life lost due to deaths from CVD occurring among members of the workforce. We have used standard procedures to make these estimates, applying age-specific mortality rates to the demographic data for the study countries. We have supplemented these calculations by referring to estimates of productivity loss attributable to disability due to CVD.

We have then gone on to consider costs relating to medical and hospital care for people with CVD. Data for these costs are difficult to procure from many countries, especially those that are still developing their health services. We have used data from each of the study countries wherever we could, but have had to be satisfied with a composite picture because not every country has the same data available.

Beside the direct costs of medical care, we have sought to develop estimates of the indirect costs of CVD. These are difficult to determine even in countries with well-developed health and social security systems so, once again, we have had only partial estimates. The costs to families of caring for people with CVD vary immensely with social custom and the extent to which publicly funded social security systems operate.

D-1. Years of potentially productive life lost

Of particular interest in the analysis of the five study countries is the potential effect of CVD on the economy, given the importance of CVD within labor force-aged cohorts. The losses are from premature death and from disability. While caution is recommended in assessing the impact of years of life lost, it is possible to estimate the impact of CVD using two measures: Potentially Productive Years of Life Lost (PPYLL) and Disability Adjusted Life Years (DALY). Costs to the economy can then be extrapolated.

A measure of productive years of life lost is most relevant to the arguments in this report because it focuses on loss among the working age population. We calculated PPYLL for the five study and two comparator countries commencing at age 35, assuming a retirement age of 65, and taking the midpoint of each group (35-44, 45-54, and 55-64) as the yardstick. By this means, each death in the first age group counted as 25 years lost (between 40 and 65), each death in the second group counted as 15 years lost, and each death in the third group counted as 5 years lost.

We applied these assumptions and the prevailing age-specific CVD death rates to the demographic projections for each country for 2000 and 2030 (we did not project to 2040 due to increasing uncertainties as the time span increases). In **Tables 6** and **7,** mortality projections assume no change in the rates of CVD or any other illness (e.g., HIV/AIDS) in each country. In the case of CVD, we have already demonstrated that without preventive interventions, risk factors and therefore CVD mortality are set to increase in most of the study countries. The numbers below are therefore underestimates.

Table 6 presents our estimates of total years of life lost due to CVD between 35 and 64 for the five study and two comparator countries for 2000 and 2030, and the death rates per 100,000 of population in that age group.

Recall also, as we explained in relation to **Table 4,** that the calculations we have made for age-specific mortality vary according to the accuracy of published mortality data. Thus when these data are incomplete, our estimates of lost productive life will be low, sometimes considerably so, compared with the real losses and those calculated on the basis of death data adjusted for under-registration and misclassification.

| | 2000 | | 2030 | |
	YEARS LOST	RATE/100,000	YEARS LOST	RATE/100,000
BRAZIL	1,060,840	2121	1,741,620	1957
S. AFRICA	302,265	2753	391,980	2667
RUSSIA	3,314,014	5684	3,208,265	5887
CHINA	6,666,990	1595	10,460,030	1863
INDIA	9,221,165	3572	17,937,070	3707
SUB-TOTAL	20,565,274		←	33,738,965
U.S.	1,631,825	1267	1,972,215	1661
PORTUGAL	40,880	1103	53,125	1317
SUB-TOTAL	1,672,705		←	2,025,340

Table 6: Total years of life lost due to CVD among the populations aged 35- 64 for the five study and two comparator countries 2000 and 2030, and the years lost rates per 100,000 (assuming current CVD rates).

Table 6 shows that the total number of years of productive life lost for the five study countries is already high and will increase from 20.6 million in 2000 to 33.7 million in 2030. Recall that we have assumed stable CVD age-specific death rates, so the increase is due solely to increasing population sizes at risk.

To gain an idea of the relative importance of CVD as a cause of lost years of economically productive life, it is helpful to look at a recent study from Johns Hopkins University, in which Zhou et al. calculated the various causes of life lost in China. They estimated that CVD accounted for 9 million PPYLL a year in China in 1998 and 1999. (57) This estimate is higher than ours (6.7 million years in 2000), perhaps for reasons to do with mortality estimates. The Johns Hopkins group assumed productive years to be from 15-64, whereas we used 35-64 and their calculations included estimates of the consequence of morbidity whereas ours did not. For comparison, Zhou et al. give a clear picture of the order of magnitude of CVD in China, with injury heading the list of lost productive life (12.6 million years), followed by CVD, cancer, respiratory disorders, and infections. Extrapolating from the Johns Hopkins study of the cost of injury in China, these PPYLL levels for CVD translate into a cost of between $6 billion and $9 billion each year. This estimate would increase in future if migration from rural areas to the cities were to grow.

Calculations made in South Africa based mortality data for 2000, as part of the initial burden of illness study in that country, indicated that CVD accounted for 848,000 years of potential life lost. The South African calculations used a wider age range than we did. CVD accounted for about 21% of potential years of life lost to NCDs. HIV was, predictably, far ahead as a cause of lost years of life, more so since 2000. (33)

Table 6 also shows that the total number of years of productive life lost for the five study countries will increase at a much greater rate between 2000 and 2030 than in the two comparator countries, even though in Brazil and South Africa the rates decrease slightly from 2000 to 2030. This is due to their anticipated demographic development.

Compared to 2000, the number of years of productive life lost to CVD will have increased in 2030 by only 20% in the U.S. and by 30% in Portugal. For Brazil the figure is 64%, for China 57%, and for India, an incredible 95%. The increase in South Africa is 28%, greater than that for the U.S. and comparable with Portugal. Only in Russia does the number of years lost lag, largely because death rates are already at such high levels and the size of the population at risk is falling.

It is instructive to disaggregate these PPYLL figures into decades for the age group 35-64 to see in which decades the changes in years of productive life lost are most significant. **Table 7** provides these data.

As one might expect, fewer years of productive life are lost in the five study countries and in the U.S. and Portugal amongst the youngest age group (35-44), consistent with the mortality rates presented for this age group in **Figure 9.** The increase in years lost between 2000 and 2030 for this age group is significant but not great, except for India, where an additional million years of life lost is anticipated (in Russia there is in fact a decrease, as there is also in the U.S. and Portugal).

2000							
	35-44	**%**	**45-54**	**%**	**55-64**	**%**	**SUBTOTAL**
BRAZIL	358,200	(34)	456,585	(43)	245,655	(23)	1,060,840
S. AFRICA	112,000	(37)	123,030	(41)	67,235	(22)	302,265
RUSSIA	975,700	(29)	1,427,190	(43)	911,125	(28)	3,314,014
CHINA	1,550,975	(23)	3,069,660	(46)	2,046,355	(31)	6,666,990
INDIA	2,260,450	(24)	3,958,995	(43)	3,001,720	(23)	9,221,165
SUB-TOTAL	**5,257,325**	**(29)**	**9,035,460**	**(44)**	**6,272,090**	**(33)**	**20,565,274**
U.S.	480,575	(29)	714,375	(44)	436,875	(27)	1,631,825
PORTUGAL	12,950	(32)	16,380	(40)	11,550	(28)	40,880
SUB-TOTAL	**493,525**	**(29)**	**730,755**	**(44)**	**448,425**	**(27)**	**1,672,702**

2030							
	35-44	**%**	**45-54**	**%**	**55-64**	**%**	**SUBTOTAL**
BRAZIL	487,550	(28)	739,695	(42)	514,375	(30)	1,741,620
S. AFRICA	124,625	(32)	156,825	(40)	110,530	(28)	391,980
RUSSIA	739,900	(23)	1,420,080	(44)	1,012,285	(33)	3,208,265
CHINA	1,767,775	(17)	3,694,530	(35)	4,997,725	(48)	10,460,030
INDIA	3,691,325	(21)	7,789,710	(43)	6,456,035	(36)	17,937,070
SUB-TOTAL	**6,811,175**	**(20)**	**13,800,840**	**(41)**	**13,126,950**	**(39)**	**33,738,965**
U.S.	442,600	(22)	740,625	(38)	788,990	(40)	1,972,215
PORTUGAL	12,300	(23)	21,765	(41)	19,060	(36)	53,125
SUB-TOTAL	**454,900**	**(22)**	**762,390**	**(38)**	**808,050**	**(40)**	**2,025,340**

Table 7: Productive years of life lost due to CVD by labor force age group in 2000 and 2030 for the five study countries and the two comparator countries, by number and percent of all years of productive life lost in each country due to CVD.

However, for the middle decade (45-54) the figures are of particular concern. Currently this decade accounts for the highest proportion of years of productive life lost for all countries, and this will remain so in 2030 for all but China and the U.S., where proportionately more years of life lost will be in the last working decade (55-64). In India, there will be almost a doubling of the years of productive life lost in this decade between 2000 and 2030, from almost 4 million to nearly 8 million. These early deaths rob the workforce of vibrant, experienced workers and families of fathers and breadwinners in mid-life. Brazil will also see a significant increase, and China and South Africa somewhat less so.

For those aged between 55 and 64, the oldest age group, productive years of life lost increases dramatically from 2000 to 2030, as countries age. Four of the five study countries will see almost a doubling of years of life lost in this age group, with China and India providing massive numbers. While Russia's increase is more modest (due to high rates already), significant increases are also expected in the U.S. and Portugal.

D-2 Disability adjusted life years lost

A second way of examining the cost of CVD is to estimate Disability Adjusted Life Years (DALY) lost. This measure includes the impact of premature mortality and disability (e.g. inability to work, prolonged illness). We have not been able to produce these figures for the five study countries because adequate morbidity data were not available to us. However, the Global Burden of Disease Study estimated that in 1990, 28.6 million DALYs were lost to CVD in India and 28.4 million in China. (26)

These numbers placed CVD among the major causes of lost DALYs, although other causes including injury and infectious diseases were more predominant. Assuming that the average income was of the order of $1000 per annum, an assumption made in the CMH Report (10), and using a low estimate of cost for each DALY lost to CVD, the costs to China and India are both of the order of $30 billion per annum. These figures are much higher than our conservative estimates of cost based on PPYLLs, and include estimates of loss beyond retirement and before age 35 years. In relation to other diseases, however, advocates have used figures determined this way to argue for investment in prevention and treatment programs that are less expensive than the imputed costs attributable to lost DALYs. Using either PPYLLs or DALYS, the magnitude of the CVD burden in China will be immense.

Disaggregated figures are not available for the other study countries. The equivalent figures for the former socialist economies were 17.1 million lost DALYs and for all established market economies, 22.1 million. (58) These figures suggest that, even in 1990, India and China were each contributing more disability-adjusted years lost to CVD than the developed world.

Information is also available for China and India on the combined healthcare system and productivity costs of diet-related chronic diseases, this category comprising coronary heart disease, stroke, hypertension, diabetes and cancer following studies by Popkin et al. While one cannot separate the costs of cancer from those attributable to the four other illnesses, the numbers are indicative. (54) The authors estimate that in 1995, the total health care costs for these five diseases (as defined above) were

$11.74 billion in China and $1.10 billion in India. The estimated productivity costs associated with premature death from these illnesses were $3.41 billion for China and $2.25 billion for India. These costs include those due to cancer. In the U.S., the authors note, total costs due to these diseases represented 3.8% of GDP in 1993, compared to 2.1% for China and 1.1% for India in 1995.

What of the impact of CVD on payrolls? Disaggregated data on CVD are available for India. It is possible to estimate costs from these data using several assumptions. For India, we assumed that two-thirds of CVD deaths are in urban areas, and used labor force participation rates by age and gender, and by urban and rural residence, to determine the distribution of deaths among working-age cohorts. We used the average industrial wage for 2001 to represent an urban wage, and halved that wage to represent a rural wage.

Applying those values to data on the distribution of CVD deaths by age and gender for the 35-64 age group in India, resulted in a total payroll loss only (not including health care costs) in a single year (2000) of $198 million. This is much the same as the annual expenditure on health care of the entire population of India over the age of 75. There is a marked urban/rural distinction. Urban areas represent 56% of the loss but 28% of the total Indian population. Because women's laborforce participation in urban India is low (25%-35%), 86% of this urban loss is attributable to male deaths compared to 73% in rural areas.

To summarize, CVD is a major cause of loss of productive years of life in developing countries and this is much more the case than in the U.S. and Portugal where the main impact of the disease occurs in older age groups. The loss of productivity is attributable both to the mortality and to the morbidity of CVD. Those responsible for macroeconomic decisions in developing countries need to consider CVD when determining their agendas.

D-3. Disability

The previous section has included a reference to disability in the commentary on DALYs. Disability studies of CVD in the workforce of industrial nations have regularly found that disability associated with hypertension and heart disease results in a large number of impaired workdays. A smaller portion of CVD death occurs in the workforce than does the portion of disability.

There are few comprehensive data available on the toll of disability associated with CVD in the developing world, either short term or long term, but CVD creates significant disability costs for both social payments and household support. China now has a stroke incidence of 1.3 million new victims per year, of whom 75% live with varying degrees of disability. (60) We can derive an understanding of the cost from data from India, Tatarstan, and South Africa.

In India, disability is on the rise. Temporary disablement benefits paid in India rose by 9% between 2000 and 2001. This measures only a fraction of disability, because only that portion of the population covered by benefits plans receives payments. If we further assume that disability precedes 5% of CVD deaths, and that the duration of disability averages three years[3], we can calculate the wage loss. The three-year wage loss for disability adds another $30 million to the CVD economic bill.

In Tatarstan, CVD accounts for 42% of all disability due to disease (as opposed to injury) in the population 18 years of age and older. While we do not have costing data, we know that CVD as a cause of temporary disability among workers has increased by 27% in the past five years, CVD disability per 10,000 people is growing by 15% per annum, and its dominance among causes of disability has strengthened.

South African estimates, from a survey reported in 1997, are that within working ages, disability increases from 6% in the 36-40 age group to 14% in the 61-65 age group. About 26% of the disability is due to illness, and 20% of that is due to hypertension, stroke and diabetes. (61) Other major causes of disability are injury, violence, pre- and post-natal conditions and poor rural medicine.

If we apply the age-specific disability rates and causes to an aging population, we can estimate the effect on the workforce of CVD-related disability. Assuming that the HIV epidemic comes under control, the number of South Africans aged 35-64 disabled by CVD will increase by 79% by 2040. The current public disability payment in South Africa is about $100 per month. Health officials have calculated that CVD accounted for 1,100,000 lost DALYs in South Africa in 2000 (33). One year's disability payments for the 2000 CVD disabled workforce would be about $70 million. By 2040, the combination of population aging and rising CVD disability with age, together with a 4% simple compound annual inflation rate, will boost that payment in real terms to about $600 million for the 35-64 aged workforce, eight times its 2000 value **(Figure 16).**

---

[3] These are extremely conservative assumptions since stroke alone represents a quarter of circulatory disease deaths and CVD itself represents 12% of hospital admissions even in rural areas.

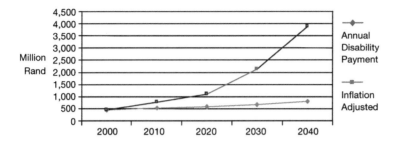

Figure 16: Annual value of disability payments (7Rand = U.S.$1) for CVD in South African workforce aged 36-65 on a current and inflation-adjusted basis.

Source: World Development Indicators 2003 (31), CASE Survey of Disability for the South African Department of Health (61)

As developing countries grow wealthier and want to do more for their people, disability payments will increase and become an increasing budgetary burden.

D-4. Direct health care costs

Several studies in the industrialized world have attempted to estimate the direct health care costs of CVD and its clinically expressed risk factors. All have found CVD to be a major driver of rising health care costs. Indeed, a study in Finland indicated that, even when CVD mortality rates fall, costs remain nearly static, in part because technological options for postponing mortality are themselves increasingly costly. (62) In the U.K. in 2000, the calculated annual direct costs of care for patients with ischemic heart disease (one manifestation of CVD) were £1.1 billion, with the indirect costs of loss of productivity three to four times greater. (63)

Estimates of the direct costs of CVD and its precursors are useful primarily in giving a sense of the enormity of the burden of these conditions on Western health systems. Thompson and Wolf in 2001 reviewed studies on the medical-care cost burden of obesity, which contributes to CVD as well as to diabetes, cancers, gall bladder and musculoskeletal problems. In a range of Western countries, obesity was estimated to contribute between 2% and 7% of total health expenditures. The higher figure refers to the U.S., and translates into a cost in 1995 dollars of $70 billion. (64) Thompson and Wolf cite estimates by the American Heart Association suggesting that the annual direct health costs of CVD are likewise enormous. The Association estimates that in 1995 dollars, coronary heart disease cost $50.8 billion, stroke $18.1 billion and hypertension $15.6 billion. The American Diabetes Association has estimated the direct costs of diabetes at $91.8 billion in 2002 of which a major portion is due to CVD. (65)

Hoffman et al. surveyed the prevalence of chronic conditions (including hypertension, diabetes and other precursors of end organ CVD) in the U.S. (66) While figures are not limited to CVD, two aspects of their findings are relevant to the consideration of CVD health costs. First, chronic conditions – compared to acute health episodes – accounted for a disproportionate share of health care expenditure, through hospital admissions, length of stay, drugs and visits to physicians. Second, when the health care costs of chronic conditions were calculated, half the estimated annual $272 billion bill came from those aged 18–64 (i.e. those of working age). These figures point to the pressures that health systems in developing countries will experience if the incidence of CVD (and other chronic conditions) is not controlled.

Myocardial infarction, acute coronary syndromes, and chronic angina absorb resources, both private and public, in those societies that can and want to treat them. Expensive high tech procedures (cardiac catheterization and coronary and peripheral angioplasty, drug eluting stents, implantable defibrillators, coronary, carotid and peripheral vascular surgery) can prolong life and enhance its quality. If pressure to embrace new technology increases in developing countries, which with global information networks it will, these countries will bear heavy economic costs. At present only OECD countries offer such advanced services and few do so on demand.

Current direct health care costs for CVD in the developing world are likely to rise as prevalence rises, and, even if rates plateau, costs are likely to become increasingly sticky as technological options spread. A study of CVD costs in South Africa from 1991 estimated that direct health system costs for CVD totaled between $230 million and $300 million. (67) This equates to between about $350 million and $470 million in August 2003 values, assuming a 4% inflation rate. This is likely to be an underestimate, since CVD rates and/or CVD expenditures per capita will have increased in the intervening 12 years.

The average cost of hospital treatment of a CVD patient (based on a South African insurance sample described above) illustrates the relative importance of CVD within the cost structure of inpatient care. On average, insurance payments for CVD inpatient care involved a modest average length of stay of three days, although the overall length of stay in all types of hospitals was up to twice as long in central hospitals in towns than in South Africa's provinces. However, the cost per admission for CVD was two to three times the average cost in a tertiary care hospital, and six to seven times the average cost of an admission in a regional or district hospital. CVD treatment costs escalate not necessarily because CVD patients are in hospital longer, but because resource consumption for CVD patients is much more intense than for the average patient. Costs per bed day were six times those of the average patient in a tertiary hospital and 10 to 15 times those of an average patient in a district or regional hospital. (67)

We calculated that in Rio Grande Do Sul, Brazil, patients admitted for circulatory disease use 10.5% of all hospital days but 20% of costs, or $379 million dollars per annum. Data relating to hospital costs provided by our contacts suggest that the cost per hospital bed day for these patients was 82% higher than the overall mean bed day cost.

In Tatarstan, the occupancy rate for designated cardiology beds in 2002 was 99%, up from 92% in 1998, even though mean length of stay had declined by 15% since 1998. Hospitals are thus moving CVD cases faster through inpatient services, but because demand has increased, this does not translate into cost savings.

Tatarstan data also illustrate the relative cost of CVD disease management. The cost of a cardiology bed day in a tertiary hospital is six times the cost of an outpatient visit to a polyclinic. If a disease management strategy could prevent, or substantially postpone, the onset of end organ CVD, for example, by paying for four annual clinic visits instead of one admission, this would dramatically reduce in-hospital costs of CVD. Such a program could reduce the need for hospital beds and prevent a portion of CVD disability.

For China, estimates from 1998 indicate that hospital costs attributable to CVD conditions totaled over $9.6 billion, or nearly 20% of all hospital costs. (57)

Urbanization increases health care expenditures. In urban settings, access to care is often greater than in rural areas. Total patient expenditures for health services in urban areas of India are higher than in rural areas, for both hospital stays and illness treatment, and for services in both government and non-government facilities. Urban households spend more on health care than their rural counterparts do at all income levels, and, except for the poorest, this expenditure is a greater portion of urban household incomes than in rural areas. Patient expenditures are 20% higher in urban than in rural areas, even where government facilities are the locus of care.

As **Table 1** indicates, in China, India and Russia, health care spending currently represents 4 to 6% of GDP, although the SARS crisis was an expensive addition to China's health budget in 2003. In Brazil it is nearly 8% of GDP and in South Africa nearly 9%. This contrasts with the U.S., where health care expenditure is nearly 14% of GDP, with expectations for treatment of conditions such as CVD ever rising.

National expenditure figures can understate the effects of health care costs at the household level. Indian insurance data indicate that Indian households allocate between 10% and 20% of household income to health care costs. (68) Increased morbidity and mortality from expensive illnesses such as CVD will push those allocations upward. In turn, this will bleed household resources away from savings and other areas of consumption and investment.

The effects of CVD on costs extend well beyond the health sector. This is especially true for the five countries studied in this report, where there is a disproportionate impact on the labor force, and hence a greater overall economic price to pay from long-term disability and early death. A 1991 study in South Africa estimated that direct health care costs account for only 42% of the total costs for CVD. (69) Hence, for every dollar spent on CVD by the health system, the South African economy pays another $1.38 due to CVD morbidity and mortality manifesting in disability and lost productivity costs.

The study of coronary heart disease in the U.K. already referred to found that the employment and other costs of informal care provided by the family for CVD patients were almost four times the size of direct health care costs. Similarly, in Switzerland, Canada and the U.S., the employment and indirect costs surpassed the costs of direct health care. (63)

D-5. Household viability and dependency

As noted in the earlier discussion of widowhood, death of the breadwinner affects the future of an entire household. This is true whether the individual dies of HIV/AIDS, an accident or CVD. Using the mortality and employment data from India, and assuming an urban household size of 5.8 and a rural household size of 5.5, we calculated that CVD deaths among the 35-64 age group affect as many as 5 million members of Indian households. (68) A study in Bengal found that when there is an adult death in a household, a child of less than two years has a 12-fold higher probability of death. (43)

Some elements of the impact of CVD on households are not easily measured, but their consequences hint at the seriousness of the trends. When members of an extended family are disabled, there are few systems of care available in developing countries. The disabled reside with their families. Frequently, young girls provide necessary care, often at the cost of their schooling. The developing world overall has made great strides in recent years in expanding young girls' schooling and women's literacy overall. In two-thirds of the developing countries surveyed by UNESCO, female literacy will exceed 75% by 2005. However, if young girls are withdrawn from school to care for disabled adults or to pursue menial labor to supplement the household incomes of their widowed mothers, this chain of success will be broken, with consequences that extend far beyond the classroom and the hospital ward.

Evidence from Tatarstan confirms that disability indeed disrupts households. In 2002 among the working population, the second most important stated reason for disability payments to the working population was "looking after patients." Taking care of someone who was ill was second only to being ill with respiratory diseases, as a trigger for being off work temporarily (with its productivity impacts) and for receiving direct disability payments. These caretaker roles represented 16% of the entire temporarily disabled population whose disability was attributable to disease. As disability rises, therefore, its economic effect will be magnified, since disability will also pull caretakers from both employment and education.

CVD deaths among working aged males also impact on households because of trends in dependency. Three quarters of India's elderly are economically dependent on their children. Over 86% of urban elderly Indian women are fully dependent on their children. Over 90% of India's urban elderly live with their families, and the portion is nearly as great in rural areas. (38) As the population ages and the dependency rate again rises, but this time skewed toward the old rather than the young, the impact of the early death of wage earners will be profound, with extensive repercussions on household viability and elderly women.

As indicated in **Figure 3** above, between 2000 and 2020, dependency will fall in all five study countries as birthrates fall. But the opportunity this creates is only a window, and like all open windows, it will close. Ultimately, dependency will rise as the number of older persons increases. Then, however, their nature will be fundamentally different to the dependency that characterized the last thirty years. **Figure 17** illustrates this change.

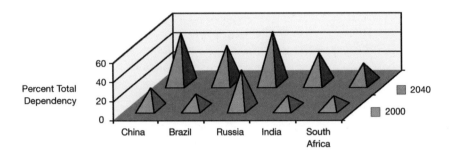

Figure 17: Percentage of total dependency attributable to the 65+ population, 2000 and 2040, in the five study countries.

Source: World Development Indicators (31)

The dependants will not be children; they will be people aged over 65. The proportion of the population under the age of five years will be less than the proportion over 65, so the proportion of dependency attributable to those aged 65+ will rise. A dependent elder is clearly not equivalent to a dependent child. Older people incur more health care costs. In industrialized countries, health care for those over the age of 65 is three times as costly as for those under the age of 65, and for people over the age of 80, three times again as expensive as for those under 80. Dependency in old age also exacts other economic costs including social security payments, increasing probabilities of disability, and increasing needs for investments in technologies that enable older people with disability to perform acts of daily living.

This coming tide of elder dependency casts the current CVD problem in the developing country workforce in a harsh light. Just at the time when developing countries' economies have the opportunity to invest more of their capacity because a brief window of lower dependency has opened, the workforce that nations count on to exploit that opportunity is itself prematurely dying.

To summarize, the costs of CVD are incurred both among mid-life and older adults. In developing countries, CVD is a potent cause of death and disability among working age people. It will become a major cause of disability among older people whose numbers are set to rise spectacularly over the next 30 years. Although in countries where HIV/AIDS is rife (such as South Africa) it is the outstanding cause of lost years of productive life, in other countries CVD and injury compete for this dubious distinction.

Because of the impact of CVD on productivity, and because of the costs of managing it and its complications, it deserves the lively interest of those charged with making macroeconomic and other economic decisions especially in middle-income countries, including those who manage the budgets of health ministries and departments.

E

Intervention strategies to reduce the impact of CVD

In contrast to the grim news about its frequency and social and economic cost, the good news about CVD is that we can do much to prevent and ameliorate it. Those interested in this goal can assess the merits of different forms of prevention, their costs, and their political and economic feasibility. They can relate them to estimates of costs of CVD and its management, and apply them as they see fit.

The terminology about prevention is confusing and it is important for us to clarify it before we proceed. This confusion is because public health practitioners and clinicians use the same name – primary prevention – for different things.

Prevention can seek to rid a society of CVD so that in a long life CVD does not ever present as a clinical problem. Public health professionals usually call this primary prevention. It implies the eradication of the primary causes of CVD, that is, of the conditions that produce the risk factors that predispose people to arterial disease.

Alternatively, prevention can aim to postpone the presentation of CVD from young or middle adulthood to old age. This enables individuals to live a full life, participate in the workforce, and experience a healthy old age, prior to the clinical onset of disease. It seeks to reduce risk factors for this purpose. Public health practitioners refer to it as *secondary* prevention. However, the clinical literature often calls this *primary* prevention.

To avoid this confusion we refer to the prevention that aims to lower the levels or eliminate risk factors as *community-based prevention* and the clinical treatment of people with elevated risk factors or expressed CVD as *clinical treatment and prevention.*

When OECD countries have brought CVD under control, they have used these preventive approaches in combination. Declines in CVD mortality have run in parallel with decades of decreasing consumption of animal fat, decreasing tobacco consumption, and growing community awareness about CVD risk factors and heart health consciousness. As well, medical and surgical treatments have improved in efficacy. These range from pharmaceuticals that lower blood pressure and cholesterol to surgical interventions. Most estimates of the effects of these interventions conclude that half of the declining CVD mortality is due to community-based prevention and half to treatment. In other instances, changing macroeconomic conditions have contributed to changes in CVD risk.

However, the countries that have experienced declines in national CVD mortality have not seen the benefits spread evenly among all groups in their societies. CVD manifests a strong social class distribution, with disease concentrating among the more socially disadvantaged, even in countries that have halved overall mortality from CVD.

E-1. Levels of prevention of CVD

Broadly speaking, there are three levels at which to implement CVD prevention.

E-1a. Macroeconomic and whole-of-government interventions that affect everyone[4]

This report seeks to locate CVD within a macroeconomic context, claiming that CVD has a serious impact on workforce productivity in developing countries. We support that claim by our analyses of the effect of CVD on workforce productivity, deaths in young adults, impact on women's health, and widowhood. The financial costs amount to tens of billions of dollars a year in China and India and less in the other study countries, but are so huge as to fully justify the attention of those concerned with macroeconomic policy in middle-income countries.

There is another aspect to the macroeconomic significance of CVD, and that is what macroeconomic policy can do to contribute directly to its amelioration. CVD takes its

---

[4] In this discussion we exclude macroeconomic interventions far removed from CVD, such as policies and programs to decrease poverty, to increase the supply of food and clean water, and to improve literacy and education. All of these initiatives are associated with increasing development, and in countries with high rates of communicable diseases, with increasing health status and longevity. In the case of CVD and other chronic diseases, they are less relevant, as countries with increasing levels of CVD tend to have substantially addressed these basic questions, at least for that section of the population at risk of CVD. CVD is, in this sense, a disease of relative affluence, rather than of absolute poverty, although the two can co-exist in the same country.

origin from the societies in which it manifests, the major risks having to do with diet, tobacco, work, wealth (or lack of it), education and physical exercise. Officials would be wise to assess the health impact of all macroeconomic policies that concern diet, nutrition, agriculture, trade, education, tobacco, the physical environment, town planning and transport, on CVD.

We can consider tobacco taxation as a macroeconomic intervention because of its relation to major sources of national revenue in many countries. Prahbat Jah and colleagues have examined the economic consequences of instituting comprehensive tobacco control strategies. These strategies include an excise on the sale of tobacco to citizens. Tobacco taxation can raise substantial revenues. Jah et al. calculated that in China, a 10 percent increase in cigarette tax would decrease tobacco consumption by 5 percent. It would also increase tobacco revenue by 5 percent, 'sufficient to finance a package of essential health services for one-third of China's poorest 100 million citizens.' (70). This work sets a fine example of the way in which we can assess the macroeconomic consequences of health interventions. It gives the lie to the global myth that only rich countries can afford to introduce tobacco control strategies.

Macroeconomic interventions thus include governmental policies in a range of fields in which national treasuries have an interest, and that impact on CVD and its risk factors. They are matters that affect a country's macroeconomic agenda. They include policies and programs such as:

- tobacco production and consumption – including subsidies, taxes, advertising and control strategies, and incentives to grow crops other than tobacco;
- nutrition – including food production, processing and marketing subsidies, such as those in relation to animal or vegetable fats, and the salt content of foods;
- education – including decisions about curricula in schools (e.g. physical or drug education, nutrition and cooking)[5] and assistance in managing stress; and
- urban planning – including recreational spaces, transport systems, and city design that encourages physical interaction with the environment.

Macroeconomic interventions usually derive from ministries other than health (such as finance, transport, education or urban development), and exert their impact on non-health sectors of the population (e.g., dairy producers). They are implicitly political in nature.

---

[5] In France, nutrition education is part of the school curriculum, encouraging an appreciation of food quality rather than quantity. Food serving sizes are smaller in France than in other European countries.

An example of a macroeconomic intervention that seems to have had an impact on CVD rates comes from Poland. In the early nineteen nineties, after separation from the USSR, heart health steadily improved in Poland, in contrast to other former Soviet republics. In 1992-94, mortality from heart disease, based on official statistics, fell by 25% from a high in the decade up to 1991. (71)

The fall in heart disease deaths coincided with a switch in Poland from consuming animal fats to vegetable fats. This resulted not from health promotion initiatives, but from a government decision to cut subsidies for animal fats and impose taxes, thus raising the price of animal fats to consumers and making vegetable oils more competitive. There followed a 23% decline in the availability of animal fat products and a 48% increase in the supply of vegetable fat products.

Margarine manufacturers pushed strongly to sell products with vegetable fat in Poland. At the same time, the government opened markets to oranges, bananas and kiwi and grapefruit year-round.

Whether these dietary changes alone accounted for the entire decline in CVD mortality is unclear. Monitoring of risk factors through the two Polish MONICA centers in Warsaw suggests that between 1987 and 1992 blood pressure and female smoking decreased, but not average cholesterol levels which were already low. (21) Huge discrepancies were noted between official and MONICA ten-year average CVD mortality rates. Macroeconomic policies made it easier for Poles to consume a healthier diet. (71) Economic policy alone can sometimes help in promoting heart health, but it is most effective when combined with other social policies, information and legislation.

E-1b. Population-based interventions

Governments and other interested agencies direct health promotion interventions at broad populations, addressing the structural and behavioral determinants of health and illness. Unlike macroeconomic policies that have to do with revenue and general government outlays, these interventions have an explicit health goal. They bring awareness of the value of good health, and create pathways to it for as large a population as possible. The methods used include media projects and advocacy together with enabling social programs about how to maintain health and reduce or avoid risk. For CVD, these comprise information and other programs addressing:

- the risks of smoking, the value of smoking avoidance, excise and taxes aimed at reducing smoking uptake and intensity, restrictions on smoking in public place and smoking advertising and smoking cessation treatment;

- the causes of high blood pressure and the benefits of control strategies;
- the causes of hyperlipidaemia and dietary recommendations;
- the dangers of obesity and warnings about diabetes;
- the importance of good nutrition and physical exercise in weight control and cardiovascular health; and
- stress and strain reduction in the workplace.

An immense literature documents the steady reduction in tobacco consumption in developed countries that has followed the introduction of comprehensive tobacco control strategies involving public education, tobacco excise and tax, bans on advertising and restrictions on smoking in public transport, restaurants, bars and places of assembly. Health promotion has been essential to this process.

The recently transacted Framework Convention on Tobacco Control, adopted at the World Health Assembly in May 2003, requires signatory countries to promote public awareness using multiple communication methods. (73) Since smoking is avoidable, the habit and its initiation and perpetuation could yield to a successful combination of macroeconomic, population-based, and health worker initiatives. The rapid and full implementation of the Framework Convention on Tobacco Control and development of its protocols deserves urgent global support.

In relation to nutrition, agriculture and food production, governments have developed hundreds of policies and programs in developed countries to modify dietary consumption of fat, especially animal fat. Their potential for benefit is huge because they aim at the entire population, seeking to achieve small reductions in risk for everyone. The effects of these small reductions in risk can be very significant when multiplied across entire populations. (72) For example, Oster and Thompson estimated that a reduction in dietary saturated fat of between only 1-3% in the U.S. would reduce coronary heart disease events by 30,000-90,000 a year, thus avoiding between $4.1 billion and $12.7 billion in medical and productivity costs.(75) *The World Health Report 2002* (Chapter 5) uses published evidence to assess a wide range of health promotion interventions highly pertinent to CVD. The chapter carefully presents the costs and imputed benefits of these programs. The analyses should prove useful to countries concerned to invest wisely in achieving control over CVD. (11)

From Finland comes a major example of population-based dietary interventions that have had beneficial effects on CVD prevalence, although in ways perhaps not originally anticipated. Finland experienced high death rates from heart disease after World

War II. Public concern about the frequency of heart attack deaths led to a regional experiment to prevent them, the North Karelia Project, which began in 1972. Because of the association of high serum cholesterol levels and heart risk, cholesterol in the diet was one of the major targets of the prevention program. Puska et al. developed a series of community-based strategies designed to change dietary behavior. These included media campaigns, collaboration with the food industry and agricultural policy changes. (77)

The initial impact was a decrease in CVD incidence in the North Karelia region compared to a control region. However, the differences between the two regions—and between North Karelia and the rest of Finland—decreased after the first five years, mainly because people in the control region also changed their behavior, to the benefit of the entire country. As dietary preferences changed, the food industry perceived new opportunities and developed products with less oil. Agriculturalists developed a new type of rapeseed plant that grew well in the cold northern climate of Finland. The local rapeseed oils sold well and cooking with vegetable oil became popular in Finnish kitchens, so that the market proportion of unsaturated to saturated fats increased. Salt reduction was also adopted by food producers. The availability of products lower in salt and saturated fats made it easier for people to comply with health messages. As stated, observers noted that many of the changes seen first in North Karelia occurred subsequently in the rest of Finland. (77)

The examples of North Karelia and Poland demonstrate the ability to change diet through macroeconomic and health promotion interventions. The evidence in relation to population-based dietary interventions to reduce CVD is nonetheless mixed. Regional population-based CVD control programs in the U.S. have not been very successful. (74) A critical appraisal of community based interventions by Ebrahim and Smith in 1997 was not encouraging. (78) Puska et al. reviewed over 50 community-based interventions that have ameliorated CVD in developed countries for their applicability in low- and middle-income countries. (62) They accept others' reviews that these programs have had a limited effect on the target risk factors, but they question whether the evaluative studies have been large enough to detect small changes. They also ask whether the extent of the intervention (the dose), compared with the massive advertising budgets of the food industry, has been anywhere near large enough to effect substantial change. For programs to succeed, Puska et al. mention the necessity of community endorsement, adequate intensity of intervention, corroborative national policy development, evaluation, and where warranted, generalization and international sharing.

Since 1986 the WHO has been sponsoring the Interhealth Programme (Interhealth Steering Committee) in China, Africa and Chile, aimed at non-communicable disease amelioration through population-based efforts in developing countries. Few hard data are available from these projects and no economic analyses. Popkin et al. reviewed efforts made in China through the 1993 National Council for Food Reform and Development to achieve a healthy national diet through changes in food production. (79) Mauritius has used nationwide programs since 1988 that have employed price, policy and educational efforts along with community education and changes in the composition of cooking oil from palm to soy. Although obesity increased slightly over the first five years of the program, other CVD risk factors including blood pressure, cholesterol, smoking and lack of exercise all changed favorably. (80)

Serum cholesterol increases as diets change in developing countries, although the dynamics of agriculture and food production differ from country to country. Kim, Moon and Popkin describe the rapid nutrition transition observed in South Korea since the 1970s and present a detailed analysis of the social environment and nutritional behavior of South Koreans over the period of interest. Although there has been a large increase in the consumption of animal products and a fall in cereal intake, fat intake has not increased markedly and obesity rates have not risen as much as in similar countries. Government-directed national efforts towards maintaining elements of the traditional Korean diet, which is lower in fat and has generous portions of vegetables, together with widespread instruction in healthy cooking, are credited with the benefits. The authors suggest that other developing countries might learn powerful lessons from South Korea. (81)

Nutritionists and economists have estimated the costs and benefits of mandatory labeling of all prepackaged food with nutritional information food labeling. They predicted in 1994 that labeling would save the U.S. $4.2 billion over 20 years through health gain at a cost of $1.5 billion. The health ministry in Canada calculated that labeling would save the country $5.3 billion in direct and indirect health costs over 20 years, at a cost of $300 million to industry. In Australia and New Zealand, mandatory nutrition labeling is projected to prevent 400 deaths a year, with savings to the health system between $47-$67 million.[6]

---

[6] An excellent analysis of the value of food labeling is to be published shortly: Hawkes C. Nutrition Labelling and Health Claims on Foods: the Global Regulatory Environment. Geneva: World Health Organization, 2004, in press

When we evaluate population-based macroeconomic and health promotion approaches to changing smoking and diet we can rarely use randomized control trials that are used to assess new medical interventions. For this reason, causal relationships are difficult to establish. And yet, in the developed world, associations among reductions in smoking, animal fat intake, salt and excess carbohydrates, and reduced rates of CVD mortality, are persistently found. These are so notable that many governments continue to embrace strategies that reduce exposure and attempt to influence individual behavior, and the WHO continues to include these strategies as an important and cost-effective element in comprehensive prevention initiatives. (76)

E-1c. Provider-based prevention

As risk factors accumulate and become more prominent in the population, CVD prevention must shift to be more individualized and medical. Interventions include the treatment and counseling of individuals in relation to risk factors such as smoking, hypertension, hyperlipidemia, diabetes, and obesity. The more risk factors a patient has, the more intense and expensive prevention of end-organ CVD becomes. In many instances, health authorities have developed clinical practice guidelines that specify best practice for the management of patients at high risk or with established disease. The treatment of risk factors, as indicated, constitutes prevention or postponement of end organ CVD.

Trials of therapy begun once overt end organ disease expression has occurred also demonstrate strong benefits for patients following myocardial infarction, the onset of congestive heart failure, or the onset of renal insufficiency. (82-87) In practice, however, reducing risk in the clinical setting is not straightforward. In the 1999 EUROASPIRE II study of 5000 patients in 15 European countries treated in hospital for ischemic heart disease, unhealthy lifestyles and high levels of risk persisted, with 22% of patients still smoking years later, 30% with a body mass index greater than 30, and 49% with blood pressure over 130/90 mm of mercury. (88) Clinicians can slow the rate of progression of early coronary or cerebrovascular disease or congestive heart failure by medical and surgical intervention. Moreover, we know that a combination of medicines and behavior modification can prevent much of the end organ damage of diabetes. Results from clinical prevention trials of pharmacological treatment for hyperlipidemia show a substantial reduction in both ischemic heart disease and cerebrovascular disease in those at high risk (83)

Hypertension is a precursor to 62% of strokes, 49% of coronary disease, and 75% of congestive heart failure. (89) While hypertension is an appropriate target for all three types of prevention, once established it is most responsive to pharmacological intervention. Analyses of 316,000 men observed for years during the multiple risk factor intervention trial known as MRFIT in the 1980s, showed strong graded relationships between serum cholesterol above 4.65 mmol per liter (or 180 mg/deciliter), systolic blood pressure above 110mm Hg, and diastolic blood pressure above 70 mm Hg, and mortality due to CHD. (90) MacMahon et al. carried out a meta-analysis in 1990 of nine major observational studies of 420,000 patients and found that a sustained 10mm Hg lower diastolic pressure was associated with 56% fewer cerebrovascular disease events and 37% fewer coronary events. (91)

Using an observational database of one million adults, Lewington and colleagues showed a profound impact of blood pressure on cerebrovascular deaths, coronary deaths, and other CVD for men and women of all ages down to a level of 115/75 mm Hg. (92) In a recent analysis from an Asian and Pacific cohort study conducted in the age groups <60, 60-69, and >= 70 years, Lawes and colleagues showed that if systolic blood pressure were 10mm Hg lower, the epidemiologically-expected mean reduction in risk of stroke would be 54%, 36% and 25% respectively at these ages, and the risk of IHD would be reduced by 46%, 24% and 16% respectively. (93)

In 1990, Collins *et al* found in an analysis of 14 unconfounded trials of anti-hypertensive drugs (chiefly diuretics or beta-blockers) that the reductions in stroke were close to those predicted from the observational studies (33-50% in trials, and 35-40% in observational studies) but less so for heart disease (2-22% in trials; 20-25% in observational studies). More recently, Law, Wald, Morris and Jordan published a meta-analysis of 354 randomized controlled trials of blood pressure lowering agents relating blood pressure to CVD risk and showed that different categories of drugs are equally effective and their effects are additive. (95)

A workshop convened by IC Health in October 2001 considered the question of how to achieve control of high blood pressure in developing countries. (96) The workshop concentrated on the need for research for this purpose. In brief, the workshop proposed a randomized community-based trial in which the study team applied the intervention, located in the primary health care setting, to 13 of 26 communities. The intervention would raise community awareness, provide education for health service providers, and dispense patient education. It would use cost-effective prescribed medications. The trial would run for two years and be evaluated using community surveys before and after the trial.

As a starting point for treating individuals with elevated risk factor levels, hypertension has much to commend it. A clinician can enter an individual's world through this door. Hypertension is easy to identify and universally recognized as a determinant of risk. Beyond the individual, the clinician can use the measurement of blood pressure to recruit families to broadly based prevention programs. The clinician can then add other treatments as necessary.

Hyperlipidemia plays a causal role in 36% of coronary disease and 18% of cerebrovascular disease as well as important roles in renal and peripheral arterial disease. (89) In MRFIT, there was a five-fold increase in coronary mortality between the lowest and highest decile of total cholesterol. (90)

Individual assessment of cholesterol level is expensive because it involves blood tests and individual patient access to them. Because of its responsiveness to dietary manipulation, hyperlipidemia is an appropriate target for all three types of intervention. However, research suggests that it is especially sensitive to pharmacological intervention. (97)

A meta-analysis of the major trials, using statins that were less potent than those are that are now available, showed a 30% reduction in major coronary events and a 20% reduction in all cause mortality, with similar benefits for men and women and old and young patients. An average reduction of 1.8 mmol per liter in low density lipoprotein C (a form of cholesterol) in populations would reduce coronary events by 60% and strokes by 17%. (98)

To simplify the management of individuals who require medication for CVD, Wald and Law recently proposed a combination pill (Polypill). It would contain three drugs (hydrochlorothiazide, atenolol, enalapril) to lower blood pressure and simvastatin for cholesterol, together with folic acid (to reduce homocysteine levels) and aspirin to inhibit platelet function. (89) Wald and Law reasoned from clinical trial data that if everyone aged 55 and over took the pill (age being the strongest predictor of CVD risk) in high-risk populations, together with younger patients at high risk or with established CVD, the Polypill could reduce ischemic heart disease events by 88% and stroke by 80%. In the U.K., which is still a high-risk population despite recent declines in CVD mortality, 96% of people who die of CVD are aged 55 and over. Wald and Law argued that treating everyone who is 55 and over (or younger if at high risk) is therefore justified, without measuring risk factors before treatment or monitoring the effects of treatment. The intention is to shift the distribution of the principal risk factors in the population, reducing the population mean value for each and reducing the risk of the entire ('sick') population. (72). They estimated that one third of people over 55 taking the Polypill would benefit, gaining an additional 11 years of life free of ischemic heart disease events or stroke. The 'number (of patients) needed to treat' to achieve a substantial benefit was thus just three. The estimated rate of side effects was 10% but serious consequences would be much rarer.

As commentators including Rodgers have suggested, we now need trials of the Polypill in different settings. (99) We need observations of the consequences of drugs in combination. Data drawn from clinical trials are among the best available to guide clinical practice but the conditions of the trials, both the patients selected and the treatment settings, may be difficult to replicate in practice. In the developing economies in this report, the age proposed by Wald and Law to begin treatment may be too high. Clinicians and others have to tailor programs to the cultural sensitivities of the population, conduct pilot studies, and establish health care delivery and distribution systems. (100) The community-based trial of blood pressure treatment proposed by IC Health (referred to earlier) might lend itself to such investigations.

Obesity is now a worldwide epidemic, with massive increases in prevalence in countries of many different levels of development. This has led to a surge in the incidence of the metabolic syndrome, which often precedes diabetes, and to the recognition that in younger individuals this leads to a more rapid development of CVD endpoints. A recent U.S. survey estimated that the age-adjusted prevalence of the metabolic syndrome was 23.7%. The findings in other societies are no more comforting. (101, 102)

Clinicians have shown that the metabolic syndrome is reversible. (2,3) Weight loss and change in fat intake can abolish insulin resistance, hypertension, hyperlipidemia, and the other metabolic disorders that define this syndrome. (3) Diabetes prevalence falls following weight loss and dietary change. Tuomilehto et al. showed that lifestyle changes in a middle-aged Finnish diabetic population led to a reduction in the prevalence of diabetes by 58% over four years. (101) The average weight loss was 4.7%. We know that reducing the prevalence of diabetes also reduces the risk of CVD. For example, the landmark U.K. Prospective Diabetes Study, carried out in the 1970s and 1980s showed that drug control of diabetes led to a reduction in complications, such as CVD. (82,83)

The impact of weight gain on the incidence of diabetes is profound. Estimates of increasing risk of diabetes over ten years for a one-kilogram increase in weight range from 4.5% to 12%. (103) In the Nurses Health Study, over 90% of type II diabetes appeared to be preventable if the nurses maintained healthy body weight and attended to lack of exercise, poor diet, smoking, and abstinence from alcohol. (104) The absolute risk for a major coronary event in a person with diabetes without known coronary disease is nearly as high as that of a person without diabetes who has established heart disease. (105)

Changing diet following heart attack may confer a benefit. The Lyon Diet Heart Study compared a Mediterranean diet to a prudent Western diet in patients who had survived a first myocardial infarction although the results of this study are in question. The authors said that the diet reduced death, non-fatal myocardial infarction, and various other endpoints, including stroke over the four-year follow-up period. (106)

Two post myocardial infarction trials, one in India and one in Britain, have also demon-strated beneficial outcomes based on dietary advice. (107,108) The Indian study randomized patients to increased fruit and vegetable consumption and a low fat, weight loss diet and showed a reduction at one year in cardiac events in the fruit and vegetables group. The Framingham Study had earlier observed the independent value of dietary fruit and vegetables. (109) The British study looked at three regimens— fat reduction, enhanced fish intake, and increased fiber. Only the high fish diet was effective in reducing all-cause mortality over two years. These examples, however, may overestimate the effect of short-term dietary interventions. Two recent reviews of dietary intervention to prevent CVD concluded that modest changes are possible, but that long-term sustainability of effect is unproven. (110, 111)

Tobacco is widely recognized as the single most important risk factor for chronic dis-eases of various kinds (including CVD). In MRFIT, smoking of up to 26 cigarettes a day tripled the risk of ischemic heart disease. (90) Smokers develop coronary events a decade earlier than non-smokers do, and patients with heart attacks who resume smoking are four times as likely as those who stop to sustain a second one. Smoking increases worker absenteeism and reduces productivity, both of which improve following cessation. (112) CVD reduction is one among many powerful arguments that have led to successful tobacco control strategies in many different countries and to recent concerted international action. Tobacco's reach is far beyond CVD, playing major roles in cancers and lung disease. (113) Smoking is responsive to all three types of intervention although macroeconomic and health promotion initiatives tend to be most effective.

Nonetheless, while concentrating on prevention, we note that the effects of smoking cessation are strong and immediate, and clinicians need to build smoking cessation into clinical risk reduction. Clinicians should urge all people who smoke to quit and assist them in doing so to reduce their chances of CVD. Those at elevated risk because of age or other risk factors should receive the most energetic and support- ive encouragement to quit. National tobacco control, which is particularly effective in preventing tobacco smoking uptake, is critical for future generations. However, it is also much easier for a smoker to quit when there are social restrictions on smoking and a prevailing attitude that favors not smoking.

E-2. Practicalities of CVD prevention

Policies for people at low risk of CVD seek to diminish or avoid tobacco use, to favor the production and use of vegetable oils over animal fats, and to encourage physical activity especially in urban areas. The goal is to alter the factors that determine neg- ative behavior patterns within the population of those not yet at risk or at minimal risk. However, high-risk patients will also benefit from these policies, finding it easier to change their behavior if there is social support for so doing.

Once there is clinical evidence of markedly elevated CVD risk factors, treatment is required. High-risk groups require more resources for prevention per person than do large-scale interventions with those at lower risk. The economics of these two approaches are not straightforward, however. A low risk group, being large in number, can rapidly multiply an intervention of low unit cost to create a large total cost. About half of all CVD mortality occurs among those with lower levels of identifiable risk and it is to this population that health promotion addresses its efforts. The 10% of the population who have the most risk factors for CVD contribute less than 50% of dis- ease events including death from ischemic heart disease.

Primary health care is the form of health care delivery preferred for the secondary pre- vention of CVD, a preference based on both equity and efficiency. The CMH Report refers to primary health care as close-to-client services (10). Primary care provides local health services to communities, and is essential for high-quality management and clinical prevention of most illnesses. In comparison to the low cost of a primary health care infrastructure (including, where necessary, drug therapies), the expense of comprehensive medical and surgical interventions to treat established end organ CVD is very high. The authors of Chapter 6 of *the World Health Report 2003* – the chapter dealing with the neglected NCD epidemics including CVD – make a strong case, which we support, for using primary health care to meet the needs of those with NCDs as well as communicable diseases. This includes the ongoing care of HIV patients receiving antiretroviral therapy. (76)

It is important to emphasize, lest there be any misunderstanding, that the conquest of CVD does not require multiple, independent, free-standing hospital facilities. Most medical problems are best served by a stable and adequately funded primary care system. Primary care is a desirable method for organizing health services for multiple purposes, and while its pedestrian appearance means that it is not attractive to donors and others who wish to identify their gifts with tower block hospitals and electronic devices, it nevertheless represents excellent value for money.

Sophisticated hospital services for CVD in developing countries are generally limited to those who can pay. It would be unfortunate if the provision of services for those with the capacity to pay distracted attention or resources from establishing first-line primary care capacity to manage CVD risk for whole populations.

The provision of services for those at elevated risk through primary care is, like the provision of antiretroviral drugs to patients with HIV, a lifelong commitment. CVD control programs are for the long haul and in committing to them, no government or interest group should think otherwise. Clinical prevention aimed at high-risk individuals requires an enduring, life-long, relationship between the patient and the person treating them, unlike single or discrete repetitive interventions such as vaccination or treatment for short-term illness.

Besides drug costs, infrastructure and management systems are important components of clinical secondary prevention programs. A comprehensive primary care service depends on a distribution system for the supply of diagnostics, pharmaceuticals and educational materials. The treatment of CVD risk factors also requires trained personnel, simple screening tests and cheap and effective interventions.

Components include:

1. A stable government and a civil society creating a context in which it is safe to visit a clinic and where disease and medical disorders are free of stigma and individual blame;
2. A national/regional/urban primary care system, together with equitable financial arrangements for care;
3. Public educational programs available in both print and other media;
4. A national and regional supply distribution system for diagnostic tests and medications;
5. Enough trained health professionals to do the work and continuing education for all of them;

6. Reliable, affordable, and predictable access to effective medications;

7. A referral system for those with clinically expressed end organ disease that may require hospital or special care.

Almost as a parenthetic comment, we note that there is another important aspect of clinical prevention to keep in mind. That is the natural history of deferred CVD. In the U.S. from 1979 to 1999, falling IHD mortality accompanied an increase of 155% in hospital admissions for congestive heart failure (CHF), which is a long-term sequel of IHD. (114) CHF is now the most common cause for hospital admission among older people and is an emerging epidemic.

E-2a. The costs of clinic-based risk factor interventions

What would a basic, first-step clinical intervention program look like and what would it cost? It is extremely helpful if a country has a publicly funded primary care clinic system as the starting point for clinical interventions directed against CVD. This provides an excellent base for the detection and recruitment to treatment of those at high risk. It can also serve as a springboard into the community to boost health promotion initiatives, which can address both social structural impediments to heart health (local attitudes to smoking, provision of adequate recreational space) and individual behavioral determinants (attitudes towards nutrition, obesity, tobacco smoking).

The World Health Report 2002 addressed the costs of clinic-based risk factor interventions and provided a range of extremely helpful analyses relating the evidence of effectiveness in relation to probable costs in a range of countries. (11) Contrary to expectations perhaps, many of the interventions yield an excellent return on investment. The authors of Chapter 5 of the Report modeled the cost and benefits of intervening with individuals whose risk of a CVD event in the next decade was 5%, 15%, 25% and 35%. Clinicians would treat individuals with drugs to lower blood pressure and cholesterol, and aspirin (unless contraindicated). A clinician would check each patient medically four times a year and a health educator would meet each patient at least once a year. Those managing the patients would perform annual laboratory tests. Health managers would link the clinical preventive approach to population-based strategies relating to tobacco, exercise and diet (including salt). The authors concluded that treating all individuals with a 35% risk was highly economically efficient, those at 25% risk was at least cost neutral and possibly efficient, and that in most places treating people even with a 5% risk made economic sense.

They said: *The most attractive strategy among all those evaluated [is] the combination of salt reduction at a population level through legislation or voluntary agreements, with health education through the mass media focusing on blood pressure, cholesterol and body mass, plus the implementation of an absolute risk approach [the 35,25,15,5% proposal just described] to managing CVD risks. (11)*

We endorse this general approach. In the basic version we propose, doctors or other health workers would measure the blood pressure of everyone who uses health clinics for any reason at all —upper respiratory infection, arthritis, or well-baby check up. They would invite patients identified as hypertensive to participate in a risk factor modification program of which smoking cessation advice and help would be central. The clinicians would also invite family members for screening. Possibly, if finances and facilities permitted, a single, non-fasting blood drawn for sodium, potassium, blood urea nitrogen (or creatinine), cholesterol, and blood sugar would provide a more complete risk profile and permit drug therapy to be fitted to the patient's condition. By way of an example, in Tatarstan such a blood test would cost 600 rubles ($20) and in India 400 rupees ($10)[7]. We recognize that even these costs may not be tolerable in very poor countries.

In relation to the pharmacological treatment of hypertension, multiple, cheap medications are now available. Pharmaceuticals in nearly every class of drug used for CVD are now off patent. There is no need to wait for a global trade agreement.

For hypertension alone, the clinician might prescribe a thiazide diuretic and a dihydropyridine calcium-channel blocker or an angiotensin-converting enzyme (ACE) inhibitor. Thiazides and calcium blockers or ACE inhibitors would cost about $1 to $1.50 per person per week in Tatarstan, and about $3 per person per week in India. If cholesterol were also elevated, clinicians could add a statin. Statins are currently expensive in both countries ($8 per person per week in Tatarstan and more than $11 per person per week in India). However, these prices are likely to reduce over time. We estimate that a regional purchaser could negotiate price reductions of 75% now and 90% in the near future, especially as more and more of these drugs come off patent. Clinicians might also consider adding aspirin, which is very cheap, for those patients in whom it is not contra-indicated.

With the addition of more drugs to the patient's regimen the marginal gains and costs become critically important. In the U.K., Marshall has recently examined the addition

---

[7] Physicians in each country supplied the costs of these laboratory services and drugs in late 2003 (in terms of out of pocket expenses).

al benefit bought by adding drugs sequentially to achieve a reduction in CVD risk. If clinicians in the U.K. were to add simvastatin to a regimen of antihypertensive agents, $250,000 would purchase a reduction of 1.2 coronary events in those patients at a 15% five-year risk of a coronary event. The same amount of money, spent on aspirin for a much larger group of individuals at a five-year 10% risk, could prevent 30 such events. (127)

Incremental cost-effectiveness calculations are critically important in settings where money to spend on interventions is very limited and must be used to best community effect. Assuming that statins become cheaply available, the total cost for treatment using antihypertensive medications, aspirin and statins, would be about $2.20 per person per week in Tatarstan and about $4.20 per person per week in India. However, recent estimates of the cost of a Polypill suggest that, if it contained only generic drugs, it could be provided for about 25 cents a week (Stephen MacMahon, personal communication).

Some of the above costs, given the large number of individuals who need treatment, pose a major problem for many countries. This is similar to the problem facing countries that need antiretroviral therapy for patients with HIV/AIDS. Seeking external aid to achieve coverage may well be an appropriate response for many countries faced with a mounting toll of CVD.

Health service administrators and others can use available cost-effectiveness data to calculate the likely benefits that would accrue from such programs in their country. Some of these therapies, as already stated, may be outside the range of financial possibility for many citizens and governments in low-income countries. Nevertheless, they are likely to be within the capacity of affluent citizens to pay, especially those who, unless treated, might consider highly expensive treatment (including surgery) when their CVD manifests. For these individuals to pay for their own treatment may be acceptable if national health service financing recognizes the need of others for support. This is desirable for equity and achieving social justice goals through health service provision.

Two other elements of a basic clinic-based prevention program for CVD are important. First, continuing education in relation to CVD prevention for the professional staff would be essential. This need not be expensive. Local health professional associations could incorporate it into on-going professional education programs, assisted by health professionals from OECD nations and elsewhere volunteering their time.

Second, and in parallel with the intervention, a public awareness campaign would enhance enrolment and participation. The facts about CVD, and how citizens, government and the private sector can prevent and treat it, should be communicated to everyone in the communities under study using all affordable communication methods and strategies as described in the health promotion literature. Government's role as a communicator, and not only a provider of care, is critical for each country's health future. Health experts need to inform society about the growing magnitude of CVD and the factors that lead to it. Informed citizens can then press for administrative and governmental support, through policy and legislation, to assist citizens to make wise pro-health choices.

Whatever choices those responsible for health systems and macroeconomics make for CVD prevention, an essential parallel activity is outcome assessment, best conducted by independent assessors. Those implementing these programs should also measure the economic costs and benefits. National or regional programs of prevention should include enough money to measure effectiveness, say 15-20% of total program budgets. Governments and health professionals can then identify unsuccessful programs early and alter or stop them, or they can enhance successful programs and then transplant them with due adaptation to where they are needed next.

F

From analysis to action

F-1. The socio-political context: instituting change in civil societies

The preceding analyses have demonstrated the size of the problem that CVD presents both now and for the next 20-30 years, in countries that have not yet attained the levels of affluence experienced in the U.S. and similar more-developed nations. These latter countries have moved through the worst of the CVD epidemic, at least as a cause of death before age 65, although it remains a major cause of death and disability in later years. What is required in sociopolitical terms to make such an achievement likely in developing countries, beyond the technical insights that underpin prevention and treatment in their various forms?

First, a stable government and openness in the society are primary ingredients; in fact, the existence of civil society (as distinct from war, gross corruption or anarchy) is a *sine qua non* of effective interventions to improve health.

With the breakup of the Soviet Union in the early 1990s, 'civil society' was used to refer to open societies and open economies where the rule of law, popularly endorsed and enacted through democratic institutions subject to the will of the people, governed both societal and economic life. The term did not exclude any type of endeavor or institution, public or private, unless that institution operated outside of the law. More recently, the term has taken on a limited meaning to embrace that group of community-based, non-profit, non-governmental institutions or movements that engage in either service provision to communities or public advocacy. This definition explicitly excludes the private sector from the institutional mix constituting civil society because it makes profits. (116) This is not our meaning, nor do we believe it is an accurate definition of the term.

By civil society, we mean the uncoerced free association of the totality of law-abiding individuals and institutions present in open societies and open economies irrespective of their economic rationale or role. (117)

For the past few decades, peoples in every geographic region have been experiencing more open economies and more open societies. Since 1955, Freedom House has produced assessments of the progress and occasional regress of political rights and civil liberties in nations around the world. Between 1973 and 2003, the percentage of countries that are free, in the sense of there being respect for civil liberties, wide scope for open political competition, and freedom of the media, rose from 54% to 75%, and the percentage of the world's population living in free nations rose from 35% to 47%. In 1986, there were fewer than 70 elected democracies in the world; by 2002 there were more than 120. (118)

These trends present a challenge and an opportunity for the management of chronic diseases including CVD in developing countries. The challenge occurs in those societies that are not open, where reaction remains firmly in the hands of a few, where corruption is rife and the few ration information and resources as they see fit. By contrast, in civil societies, two elements create a great opportunity.

First, information is widely available, whether issued by governments, dug up by journalists, unveiled at professional meetings, or accessed on the internet. There may be questions about its quality, but not about its quantity. Second, people have the ability to organize, assemble, and speak out, and not only to do so quietly at the ballot box once every few years. An open media and freedom of assembly, together with a competitive political playing field, enable constant public challenging of anything that compromises deeply held values or hopes. Knowledge can become the motivation for the creation of new organizations (disease advocacy associations, for example), or the spur to widespread public demand for change (as the ranks of widows grow, for example). As knowledge drops into a civil society pool, the ripples of change move outward across the societal surface, touching and changing diverse sectors. (119)

Citizens and citizen groups can apply pressure to governments to create pro-health policies through taxes (such as an excise tax on tobacco) and regulations. When government in a civil society institutes such measures in response to community advocacy, it is possible to counter the argument that they are interfering with individual liberties. The restrictions, taxes, health information or other social instruments put in place are in response to pressure from an informed electorate, and not imposed paternalistically by a 'big brother' government or a 'nanny state'.

It is also true, however, that in free societies people can choose not to comply, especially where individual behavior change is concerned. In a centrally controlled political system, if the optimal programmatic solution to the erosion of health status is physical exercise, the system can mandate exercise. In an open society, policy makers can mandate to their hearts' content, but the people may or may not respond. The levers of change are no longer in the hands of ministries, but individuals. However, governments may create environments where individual pro-health decisions become easier choices, and the pressures of interests that promote unhealthy food or tobacco smoking can be restricted through government action, mandated by the electorate.

There is a final element necessary to institute change in CVD in developing countries –trust. If the public is to accept interventions that favor healthy choice and limit their freedom, through tobacco control strategies, food subsidies and pricing, trust is crucial. Society must have grounds to trust government agencies, health officials, health care professionals, academia, and the media. If the public is to trust information on different health risks (less animal fat, more fish) and treatments (medications for hypertension), the information must come from respected professionals, empowered consumer groups and professional bodies. The public must see the information as being free of political bias and of conflicted interest.

Trust also operates as governments build relationships with new partners, including business, organized labor, social security systems, and insurers, which may all be critical partners in the fight against a rising tide of chronic disease. Developing country ministries or departments of health will need to become more permeable to private initiative, which currently accounts for half of all health care resources, as well as public concern. (29,119)

What does this mean for health care systems under conditions of a growing chronic disease burden, especially of CVD, and spiraling death rates within the working age population? To the extent that civil society exists in a country, then clearly facts about CVD will become public knowledge and lead to public action, particularly among the best-informed at-risk population–urban families.

In societies with well-informed citizens, this in turn may lead to the emergence of interest groups, such as heart associations, or anti-smoking lobbies, for example. These groups represent a health system opportunity. Such interest groups and voluntary organizations, ubiquitous in civil societies in developed countries, provide both an outlet for information and public education, and a means for channeling individual concern into productive societal change. Interest groups can campaign for greater action, including support for all individuals to have equitable access to essential medications that can substantially reduce risk.

An approach that reaches from the highest levels of macroeconomic decision-making to individual citizen volition, assuming realistic responsibility for their health, has much to commend it.

Interest groups can also be important conduits by which health systems can influence other sectors of government in support of health. They can carry the message to ministries of finance and other executive offices that the public values increased resource commitments to health care. In so doing, they can influence non-health settings to consider health impacts, and can do so perhaps at times more effectively than government advocates for health care budgets. Alongside this, they can also educate the public, motivate behavior change and encourage compliance with therapeutic programs that prevent life-threatening incidents. Their presence, and their access to information and to large numbers of concerned individuals, can result in heightened demands for government responsiveness and accountability.

In relation to chronic diseases such as CVD, governments in open societies in developing countries will increasingly find themselves held accountable for reversing rising risk factor prevalence and death rates by coalitions whose constituents are most affected by CVD. The interest groups may also lobby them heavily to provide hi-tech care. The citizenry will not just generally expect accountability; it will specifically demand it. For government public health leaders, the existence of private interest groups and professional organizations dedicated to chronic diseases will result in public expectations of health policy and health service responses that are focused and articulate.

In the case of CVD, where risk factors are well recognized and a range of effective interventions available, there will be strong pressure on governments to respond. There is a growing literature on the process of translating knowledge of the environmental determinants of non-communicable disease, especially CVD, into effective health policy. In civil societies, people do choose, but unless we take care in attending to the environment, broadly defined, then healthy choices become difficult choices. (120) Part of the challenge is to provide timely and convincing information about these interventions, including the opportunity cost of intervening and not intervening, to those who are making public policy decisions day by day.

These responses require governments to move beyond the bounded notion of health systems and health departments populated by health professions who operate solely in terms of their technical expertise. There has been a tradition in developing countries that governmental public health departments focus on controlling communicable disease threats (engaging in environmental control, running mandatory immunization campaigns, isolating disease outbreaks to prevent their spread) and on improving access to clean water and healthy food. However, with chronic disease, macroeconomic decision-making and individual behavior and its social determinants are the principal concerns. In the future, public health departments will need to respond to NCD threats by participating in economic debates to help establish agendas that take due account of these health needs of the community.

Building relationships with new partners may prove difficult for some. But the need for change is also an opportunity. The opportunity allows for the building of new coalitions for health and health care that are more powerful and effective than those that exist at present. Partners who speak from the podium of business, labor, and finance can raise the visibility of health care in arenas where policy makers make decisions about fundamental economic priorities and policies. That indeed would be a novel opportunity for global health.

F-2. CVD as a macroeconomic challenge

The work of this report grew out of the work of the Commission on Macroeconomics and Health. Our argument is that in low-and middle-income countries, non-communicable diseases should be included along with communicable diseases when health is elevated to a matter of macroeconomic interest. We have shown that CVD warrants inclusion because of its immense impact as a cause of death and disability, especially among people of working age and among women. CVD hits the workforce directly and indirectly and undermines family viability in many developing countries, and these blows will fall more heavily in the future. Retired people will experience CVD as a cause of morbidity as populations age and the ranks of those aged 65+ increase dramatically in the next 20-30 years. Health services and social security systems will be especially affected.

Since the work of the CMH, many countries have expressed an interest in formulating their health policies for the future within a macroeconomic context. As indicated, several have formed their own macroeconomic commissions, as recommended by the CMH Report.

We commend our report to the attention of those many interested individuals in countries who have elected to join the WHO Macroeconomics and Health implementation program. They can do much to ameliorate CVD, but it is a race against time: strategies to reduce risk exposure and treat those at high-risk need immediate application to achieve their best effects, in the workforce now and with older citizens in the next two decades. Therefore, countries need to develop CVD control strategies now to maintain health and reduce costs. CVD control should therefore be an important part of a comprehensive macroeconomic approach to development. Economic benefits will flow from CVD prevention because of the immediate impact prevention will have on workforce mortality and morbidity.

What can prudent decision makers, such as members of a national macroeconomics and health commission who work in the ministry of health and the ministry of finance, expect to gain from a CVD prevention program? Existing cost-effectiveness and economic data, need to be refined country by country. (120) A prudent course of action would be for every civil society to examine carefully the cardiovascular health impact of macroeconomic decisions that pertain to agriculture and food production and marketing, and tobacco control. (75) Participation in international efforts to curtail tobacco consumption has been justified in multiple analyses, and one of the benefits of smoking cessation is an immediate reduction in CVD risk.

A national macroeconomic commission facing the future depicted in this report would do well to approach a long-term solution not as a problem of health care, but as a challenge in which health is intertwined with economics, education, culture, and human behavior. The old mold of public health as a health sector function must be set aside and replaced with one that sees health as a critical investment that reaches deeply into the economy and larger community to involve both the leaders and the levers with influence on the origins and solutions to the problem.

F-2a. Who should be at the table?

A national CVD effort must involve health leadership, both from public health and from the medical services professions. But also (and equally) needed at the table are:

a. opinion leaders from all levels of business, in recognition of the impact of CVD on the workforce and because some sectors (food production and sales, for example) are important for CVD control;
b. representatives from cooperatives and organized labor;
c. private financial institutions to address capital needs for health infrastructure;

d. public financial institutions (ministries of finance and central banks, since the future of labor productivity is at risk, the costs of doing nothing will be tremendous, and the policies that might be needed to alter the costs of risk behaviors are under the control of public finance);

e. social security system managers and private insurers, who will pay the direct price of disease and disability;

f. representatives of the education sector at all levels, (since prevention must start with behavior change and behavior change starts with knowledge and attitudes);

g. community groups with particular levers on the problem (women's groups, health lobby groups, athletic groups/clubs), and;

h. communications firms/agencies, whose expertise will be an asset in any effort to change opinion, attitudes and behavior.

F-2b. What should be on the agenda?

The national coalition brought together under the auspices of the national macroeconomic commission if it exists, or a similar agency if it does not exist, will need to address the CVD problem in all its dimensions, from roots to consequences. Their discussions will not always be easy, and will risk a clash of vested interests.

An agenda would first need to consider the *problem.* This would involve:

a. determining its severity and spread;

b. identifying its roots in the demography, culture and risk behaviors of that country; and

c. identifying the policies, norms and economic and social structures that support those risk behaviors.

Attention could then turn to what has been done about the problem to date, and how much success or failure has followed. There should be careful study of what the citizenry know about CVD and what they do not know and should know.

It would also be important to focus on the *vested interests* that may aid or hinder the creation of a solution to the problem. These vested interests may include competing economic priorities, private sector practices not conducive to health, health services themselves, and the structure of social security payments and the various social support systems (informal) that operate in that country. These will be difficult discussions and will raise questions of resources, costs, and burden sharing. They will require private and public collaboration and compromise. It would be desirable to enunciate all barriers, including those that are economic, that have to do with trade, that are cultural and political, and those that are due to prevailing regulatory systems.

The group should then consider the costs of not acting – in human health and economic terms. Identifying political costs both of acting and of doing nothing may also prove to be helpful.

F-2c. What resource pools do national leaders need to mobilize?

If these discussions are to be more than theoretical, those in charge of resources must put them on the table. These people must be represented in, and see themselves as co-owners of, the solution. Resources concern and include more than just health budgets. They extend to those in ministries of social security and social welfare, industry, finance, labor, youth affairs, planning, housing, and agriculture. They also extend to the private sector, both private industries and financial houses.

Philanthropy is also a potential resource. In many middle-income countries, private philanthropy is emerging as a powerful force in community development and in health and education. Domestic philanthropy (and international, to the extent that it is interested) is a pool to be assessed and involved.

Where a country receives international development assistance, the national macroeconomic commission or other responsible group should consider that as another resource. By and large, however, international development agencies do not have health assistance policies that are conducive to public-private collaboration in chronic disease control. In most cases these activities will entail a change of policy regarding the definition of health care and what constitutes health leadership. But, if a national macroeconomic commission and its opinion leaders can organize a coalition, define the problem, commit to a solution, and mobilize local resources to begin to implement the solution, bilateral and multilateral agencies will have little option but to follow. Different countries may take different approaches, combining population-based prevention and clinical prevention in unique ways. But to do nothing will put governments and their leaders in the untenable position of accepting high levels of death and disability both now and in future.

G

Conclusions

In the U.S., beginning in the 1960s with medicines of that era, diffuse public awareness programs leading to individual behavior change, and incorporating new therapeutic insights and procedures along the way, CVD mortality dropped by more than 50% in 35 years. Countries facing the challenge of an emerging epidemic of CVD could now probably do as well in half the time. Now we have better drugs that are easier to take (once a day rather than more frequently), tobacco policies that are now widely accepted, consensus-driven dietary recommendations and a recognition of the importance of physical exercise and the social origins of the CVD risk factors. There is also an understanding of the role of civil society and prudent incorporation of invasive medical and surgical procedures for those at grave risk where society can afford these.

This report poses a dramatic challenge to the public health community, to governments and private enterprise. It also challenges citizens in virtually every country. It suggests that without concerted, ongoing intervention to prevent the precursors and reverse the negative effects of CVD in developing countries, a global health crisis in the current workforces (and later among the elderly) of those countries will occur – and sooner, rather than later. Indeed, in Tatarstan this crisis is already apparent. It is also apparent in several other former Soviet states and is emerging in China, India and Brazil. This crisis hits not only individuals and their families, although this is clearly intensely important, but the economies of nations, as skilled workers die or become disabled in the prime of life, women are widowed and older people require expensive medical interventions and social support for disability related to CVD.

Yet CVD is largely a silent killer. Unlike measles, a dramatic illness that kills and maims swiftly, and where one key intervention – immunization – will prevent it, the causes and manifestations of CVD are multiple, and the progress of the disease in each individual takes years. Evidence from Western nations suggests that the negative effects of diet, and lack of exercise, for example, begin in childhood, but do not manifest as symptoms for decades.

Partly for these reasons, unlike measles, CVD has yet to take centre stage as a recognized problem in the developing world, or among international agencies that assist developing countries. In addition, CVD is seen (wrongly) as a disease only of affluence, and increasingly, of old age. All that must change, and it is beholden upon agencies and individuals who work with the populations in developing countries to include CVD in their considerations.

Combating CVD requires action on a wide range of fronts. What follows is a statement of how we propose to move forward beyond this report. This will necessarily involve research, trial interventions to assess alternative prevention and treatment regimes, consultations with governments, professionals and private industry, macroeconomic and microeconomic initiatives, and powerful advocacy of greater clarity to change individual, social, legislative and commercial behavior to make affluence less toxic in the developing world.

G-1. Putting CVD in the developing world on the international health and development agenda

We need to invest additional effort to increase recognition of CVD as an epidemic in the making, including advocating for its inclusion in the strategic priorities of international health, economic and aid agencies. To this end, we will continue to present our findings at international meetings, and to participate in global development and health initiatives where possible. As a first step, CVD and other NCDs should be included amongst focal diseases for attention through initiatives arising out of the Report of the Commission on Macroeconomics and Health, beginning with China, India, Brazil and South Africa.

G-2. Deeper documentation of the prevalence and costs of CVD

Our study has examined CVD in five developing countries, using in the main routinely available data (which are albeit sometimes hard to get, especially in the case of economic data). In order to put a persuasive case to governments concerning the need to act in relation to CVD, it is important that assessments that are more detailed be made of CVD prevalence and costs. We propose initially to do this in four countries, including South Africa and India, for which good data sets exist. This will require work in the countries by people committed to the task of data extraction. We will do this in co-operation with IC Health, which will support people in the selected countries to perform this function.

G-3. Developing partnerships at the macroeconomic level with national governments in key developing countries

We will use the data collected in point 2 above, as well as those provided in this report, as entry points to advocacy work in several developing countries. This work will aim first at putting CVD on those countries' health and development agendas, and then on establishing working partnerships with representatives in the countries to pursue policy recommendations in relation to CVD management and prevention. This will include, where relevant, health system and health delivery initiatives, and work with government agencies in relation to taxes on tobacco products, subsidies for agricultural products, food labeling, guidelines for town planning and transportation systems etc. We propose to undertake this work initially in four countries: Brazil, South Africa, China and India. In all four countries, we have established contacts.

G-4. Train the trainer initiatives in health education

Low- and middle-income countries vary in the extent to which they have trained health personnel capable of providing close-to-client primary care services. Often, educators will have trained these personnel primarily in the treatment of communicable diseases and in basic public health requirements. They may require additional training in the management of CVD. Specialist doctors and nurses will provide this training by donating their time to work with professionals on the ground in the countries concerned. Training will also include the development of treatment protocols, complementing the WHO initiatives such as the *WHO CVD-Risk Management Package* for low-and medium-resource settings.

G-5. Undertaking trial treatment and prevention interventions

There are many possible points of entry for prevention and treatment of CVD and its precursor conditions. We propose two complementary strategies. First, focusing on hypertension, we will seek cooperatively to develop treatment interventions in three or four countries. In Tatarstan and India, we could use existing polyclinics and other primary care facilities. In South Africa the establishment or reactivation of primary care facilities for the expanded programs of treatment of HIV/AIDS with antiretroviral drugs may provide a good opportunity for also treating CVD risk factors. In Brazil, with a government now committed to expanding primary care, it may be a good time to investigate what is possible for CVD treatment. In all of these countries, we will seek out industries that might be interested in supporting these approaches. U.S. multinationals (Dell, IBM, Microsoft) with large workforces in India, for example, may be willing to support these programs.

G-6. Longer term research and interventions

It is critically important to establish a research base for interventions and changes to the health systems that a CVD control program would bring. To demonstrate to governments the benefits of controlling CVD and its precursor conditions, ongoing research and evaluation in a range of countries is required. This involves working with existing bodies (such as IC Health et al.), and developing a research capacity in countries where this is lacking. The intention would be twofold: to confirm that the preventive interventions in which they have invested are producing the goods, and second, to learn from the experience and apply it elsewhere.

We are confident that this agenda will help advance CVD control in developing economies and we look forward to working with colleagues around the world to achieve this goal.

H

Acknowledgements

We gratefully acknowledge the help and contribution of individuals from various institutions who have assisted us with this report.

Dr. Jeffrey Sachs was a regular supporter and stimulating colleague who made the project happen.

Name and affiliations of external reviewers of the report

Dr. Derek Yach MD
Representative of the Director-General
The WHO, Geneva, Switzerland

Prof. John Chalmers AC MD
Professor of Medicine
The George Institute for International Health
University of Sydney
Sydney, Australia

Dr. Corrina Hawkes
Health Policy Assistant on Non-
Communicable Disease Longterm Strategy
The WHO, Geneva, Switzerland

Prof. Stephen MacMahon
Co-Director
The George Institute for International Health
University of Sydney
Sydney, Australia

Prof. K. Srinath Reddy MD
Coordinator of IC Health and Professor
of Cardiology, All India Institute of Medical
Sciences New Delhi, India

Dr. Kerr L. White MD
Formerly of the Rockefeller Foundation
and Johns Hopkins School of Public Health
Baltimore, U.S.

At Columbia University we also gratefully acknowledge the critical reading of the report by **Ms. Ann Rosenberg,** Deputy Director of the Access Program and **Dr. Paul Wilson,** Senior Task Force Associate with the Millennium Program HIV/AIDS Task Force, and **Dr. Josh Ruxin,** Director of the Macro Health Project and the Access Program, all from the Center for Global Health and Economic Development.

The Australian Health Policy Institute at the University of Sydney, the Global Forum for Health Research through the Initiative for Cardiovascular Health Research in The Developing Countries, and the Earth Institute at Columbia University through the Center for Global Health and Economic Development, all supported this project.

The contributions of the following people have included providing us with data and comments and arranging for us to meet others who have been helpful as well.

South Africa

Dr. Krisela Steyn MD
Director, Chronic Diseases of Lifestyle Unit
The Medical Research Council
Cape Town, South Africa

Mrs. Christelle C. Kotzenberg MD
Chief Director of Non-Communicable
Diseases Cluster
Department of Health
Pretoria, South Africa

Dr. Rosana Norman MD
Burden of Disease Research Unit
The Medical Research Council
Cape Town, South Africa

Dr. Debbie Bradshaw MD
Director, Burden of Disease Research Unit
The Medical Research Council
Cape Town, South Africa

Dr. Kathleen Kahn MD
Department of Community Health
University of the Witwatersrand
Johannesburg, South Africa

India

Prof. K. Srinath Reddy MD
Co-coordinator, Initiative for Cardiovascular
Health Research in the Developing Countries
and Professor of Cardiology
All India Institute of Medical Sciences
New Delhi, India

Dr. Kavita Sivaramakrishnan
Senior Research Officer, IC Health
All India Institute of Medical Sciences
New Delhi, India

Prof. K.S. Calpti Rao
Institute for Studies in Industrial Development
Narendra Niketen I.P. Estate
New Delhi, India

Geneva

Dr. Colin D. Mathers
Coordinator, Epidemiology and Burden
of Disease Global Program on Evidence
for Health Policy (GPE)
The WHO Geneva, Switzerland

Dr. Derek Yach MD
Representative of the Director-General
The WHO Geneva, Switzerland

Dr. Robert Beaglehole MD
Head, Department of Health Promotion,
Surveillance, Prevention and Management
of Non-Communicable Disease
The WHO Geneva, Switzerland

Dr. Corrina Hawkes
Health Policy Assistant on Non-
Communicable Disease Longterm Strategy
The WHO Geneva, Switzerland

Russia

Dr. Kamil Sh. Zyatdinov MD, PhD, D.Sci
Minister for Health
The Republic of Tatarstan, Russia

Dr. Vladimir G. Sherputovski MD, PhD
Head of the Republican Medical
Information Center
The Republic of Tatarstan, Russia

Prof. Ildus G. Nizamov MD, PhD, D.Sci
Deputy Head of the Kazan State Medical
Academy for Postgraduate Medical
Education, and Head of the Department
of Public Health
The Kazan State Medical Academy, Russia

Prof. Lilia E. Ziganshina MD, PhD, DSci
Chief Clinical Pharmacologist of the
Republlc of Tatarstan, Head of the
Department of Clinical Pharmacology
The Kazan State Medical Academy, Russia

Brazil

Prof. Mario Maranhao MD, FACC,
FAHA, FESC
Professor of Cardiology at Evangelic
School of Medicine and Hospital
Curitiba, Brazil
Immediate Past President of the World
Heart Federation

Prof. Aloyzio C. Achutti MD
Formerly of the Federal University of Rio
Grande Do Sul and The Academy
of Medicine from the State of Rio
Grande Do Sul
Rio Grande Do Sul, Brazil

Prof. Maria Ines Reinert Azambuja MD
The Public Health Department
The Federal University of Rio Grande Do Sul
Rio Grande Do Sul, Brazil

Prof. Carisi A. Polanczyk MD
The School of Medicine
The Federal University of Rio Grande Do Sul
Rio Grande Do Sul, Brazil

References

1. Levenson JW, Skerrett PJ, Gaziano JM. Reducing the global burden of cardiovascular disease: the role of risk factors. *Prev Cardiol.* 2002;5:188-199.

2. Mokdad AH, Bowman BA, Ford ES, Vinicor F. et al. The continuing epidemics of obesity and diabetes in the U.S. *JAMA.* 2001; 286:1195-1200.

3. Reaven G. Metabolic syndrome: Pathophysiology and implications for management of cardiovascular disease. *Circulation* 2002; 106:286-88.

4. Magnus P, Beaglehole R. The real contribution of the major risk factors to the coronary epidemics: time to end the "only-50%" myth. *Arth Intern Med.* 2001; 161:2657-2660.

5. Kuper H, Marmot M. Job strain, job demands, decision latitude, and risk of coronary heart disease within the Whitehall II study. *Epidemiol Community Health.* 2003;57(2):147-53.

6. Stamler J. The marked decline in coronary heart disease mortality rates in the U.S., 1968-1981; summary of findings and possible explanations. *Cardiology* 1985;72:11-22.

7. Thom TJ. Stroke mortality trends. An international perspective. *Ann Epidemiol.* 1993;3:509-518.

8. Dobson AJ, Gibberd RW, Wheeler DJ, Leeder SR. Age-specific trends in mortality from ischemic heart disease and cerebrovascular disease in Australia. *Am J Epidemiol.* 1981;113:404-412.

9. Ireland AW, Lawson JS. The changing face of death: recent trends in Australian mortality. *Med J Aust.* 1980;1:587-590.

10. The WHO. *Report of the Commission on Macroeconomics and Health: Investing in Health for Economic Development.* Geneva: the WHO, 2001

11. The WHO. *The World Health Report 2002: Reducing Risks and Promoting Healthy Life Geneva:* the WHO, 2002.

12. Yusuf S, Reddy S, Ounpuu S, Anand S. Global burden of cardiovascular diseases: part I: general considerations, the epidemiologic transition, risk factors, and impact of urbanization. *Circulation* 2001; 104: 2746-2753.

13. Mathers CD, Stein C, Fat Ma D, Rao C. et al. *Global Burden of Disease 2000. Version 2: methods and results.* Geneva: the WHO, 2002.

14. The WHO. *Integrated Management of Cardiovascular Risk: Report of a the WHO Meeting.* Geneva: The WHO, 2002.

15. Yusuf S, Reddy S, Ounpuu S, Anand S. Global burden of cardiovascular diseases: Part II: Variations in cardiovascular disease by specific ethnic groups and geographic regions and prevention strategies. *Circulation* 2001; 104: 2855-2864.

16. National Center for Health Statistics, CDC. (http://www.cdc.gov/nchs/fastats/heart.htm)

17. Hunink MG, Goldman L, Tosteson ANA, Mittleman MA. et al. The recent decline in mortality from coronary heart disease, 1980-1990. *JAMA.* 1997; 277: 535-542.

18. Reddy KS, Yusuf S. Emerging epidemic of cardiovascular disease in developing countries. *Circulation* 1998; 97:596-601.

19. Uemura K, Pisa Z. Trends in cardiovascular disease mortality in industrialized countries since 1950. *World Health Stat Q.* 1988; 41:155-178.

20. Bobak M, Marmot M. East-west mortality divide and its potential explanation: proposed research agenda. *BMJ* 1996; 312:421-425.

21. Tunstall-Pedoe H. the WHO MONICA Project. *J Clin Epidemiol.* 1988; 41:105-113. and MONICA Monograph and Sourcebook, the WHO, Geneva, 2003.

22. Ezzati M, Hoorn SV, Rodgers A, Lopez AD et al. and the Comparative Risk Assessment Collaborating Group. Estimates of global and regional potential health gains from reducing multiple major risk factors. *Lancet* 2003; 362:271-280.

23. Machipisa L. Women and girls carry the heaviest burden. (http://www.ipsnews.net/hivaids/section1_3.shtml)

24. Omran AR. *The Epidemiologic Transition: A Theory of the Epidemiology of Population Change.* Milbank Memorial Fund Quarterly Vol. XLIX (4); 1971:509-538.

25. Fox, DM. *Power and Illness: The Failure and Future of American Health Policy.* University of California, Press, 1993.

26. Murray CJL, Lopez AD. Alternative projections of mortality and disability by cause 1990-2020: Global Burden of Disease study. *Lancet* 1997; 349:1498-1504.

27. Kuulasmaa K, Tunstall-Pedoe H, Dobson A, Fortmann S. et al. Estimation of contribution of changes in classic risk factors to trends in coronary-event rates across the WHO MONICA Project populations. *Lancet* 2000; 355:675-687.

28. The WHO. *Diet, Nutrition, and the Prevention of Chronic Disease: Report of a the WHO Study Group. Technical Report Series 797.* Geneva: the WHO, 1990.

29. Raymond S. Foreign assistance in an aging world. Foreign Affairs 2003; 82:91-105.

30. The WHO Statistical Information System (the WHOSIS), 2003. http://www3.who.int/whosis/menu.cfm

31. 2003 World Development Indicators CD-ROM, World Bank. (http://devdata.worldbank.org/hnpstats/deaselection.asp)

32. United Nations Population Division. World Population Prospects: The 2002 Revision Population Database. (http://esa.un.org/unpp)

33. Bradshaw D, Groenewald P, Laubscher R, Nannan N. et al. *Initial burden of disease estimates for South Africa, 2000 Cape Town:* South African Medical Research Council, 2003.

34. Edwards R. Hypertension prevalence and care in an urban and rural area of Tanzania. *J Hypertens.* 2000;18:145-152.

35. Walker RW, McLarty DG, Kitange HM, Whiting D. et al. Stroke mortality in urban and rural Tanzania. Adult Morbidity and Mortality Project. *Lancet* 2000; 355:1684-1687.

36. Raymond S. *Improving People's Health. Background Paper for Foreign Assistance in the National Interest,* U.S. Agency for International Development, 2002.

37. Weir DR, Willis RJ, Sevak P. *The Economic Consequences of a Husband's Death: Evidence from the HRS and AHEAD.* University of Michigan, prepared for the Second Annual Joint Conference for the Retirement Research Consortium, May 2000.

38. U.S. Bureau of the Census, International Data Base. (http://www.census.gov/ipc/www/idbnew.html)

39. UN Demographic Yearbook, Historical Supplement 2000.

40. Haram N. Muslim widows: a case study in Delhi. *Publ Bulletin* 2002.

41. De Silva WI. How serious is ageing in Sri Lanka and what can be done about it? *Asia-Pacific Population Journal* 1994; 9:19-36.

42. Andrade M, Devos D. *An Analysis of Living Arrangements Among Elderly Women in Brazil.* presented to the Brazilian Association of Population Studies, Minas Gerais, Brazil November 2002.

43. Giri VM, Khanna M. Status of widows of Vrindavan and Varanasi: a comparative study. (http://griefandrenewal.com/widows_study.htm)

44. The UN Food and Agriculture Organization (FAO) Releases Annual Report: The State of Food and Agriculture, 2001. (http://www.rlc.fao.org/prensa/coms/2001_28.htm)

45. Researchers Call for Speeding up Urbanization in China. *People's Daily,* March 27, 2000.
46. De Melo Monte-Mor RL. *New Urban Frontiers: Contemporary Tendencies in Brazil's Urbanization,* Centro de Desenvolvimento e Planejamento Regional, 2001.

47. United Nations Environmental Program database. (http://urban.unep.net/index.php?struct_id=gurb-trend)

48. Padam S, Singh SK. Urbanization and urban transport in India: The sketch for a policy. *The Transport Asia Project,* 2001.

49. World Urbanization Prospects: The 2001 Revision. Population Division, Department of Economic and Social Affairs, UN Secretariat 2002.

50. Kahn K, Tollman SM, Garenne M, Gear JS. the WHO dies from what? Determining the cause of death in South Africa's rural northeast. *Trop Med Int Health.* 1999; 4:433-441.

51. Bradshaw D, Steyn K. *Poverty and chronic diseases in South Africa: Technical report 2001.* Cape Town: South African Research Council, 2001.

52. Singh RB, Suh IL, Singh VP. et al. Hypertension and stroke in Asia: Prevalence, control and strategies in developing countries for prevention. *J Hum Hypertens* 2000; 14:749-763.

53. Howson CP, Reddy KS, Ryan TJ, Bale JR, Editors; Committee on Research, Development, and Institutional Strengthening for Control of Cardiovascular Diseases in Developing Countries, Institute of Medicine. *Control of Cardiovascular Diseases in Developing Countries: Research, Development, and Institutional Strengthening.* Washington D.C: National Academy Press, 1998.

54. Popkin BM, Horton S, Kim S, Mahal A. et al. Trends in diet, nutritional status, and diet-related noncommunicable diseases in China and India: the economic costs of the nutrition transition. *Nutr Rev.* 2001; 59: 379-390.

55. Case study for the People's Republic of China. *Food and Nutrition Bulletin* 2001;22:34-41.

56. Piegas LS, Avezum A, Pereira JC, Neto JM. et al. AFIRMAR Study Investigators. Risk factors for myocardial infarction in Brazil. *Am Heart* J. 2003; 146:331-338.

57. Zhou Y, Baker TD, Rao K, Li G. Productivity losses from injury in China. *Inj Prev.* 2003; 9:124-127.

58. IC Health: sustainable programs for the control of cardiovascular disease and diabetes in developing countries http://www.ichealth.org

59. Kessler RC, Greenberg PE, Mickelson KD, Meneades LM. et al. The effects of chronic medical conditions on work loss and work cutback. *J Occup Environ Med* 2001;43:218-225.

60. China CVD Statistics. American Heart Association 2001. (http://www.essentialdrugs.org/newsview.php/63)

61. Community Agency for Social Enquiry (CASE), Pretoria: Survey of Disability for the South African Department of Health, 1997

62. Kiiskinen U, Vartiainen E, Pekurinen M, Puska P. Does prevention of cardiovascular diseases lead to decreased cost of illness? Twenty years of experience from Finland. *Prev Med.* 1997; 26:220-226.

63. Liu JLY, Maniadakis N, Gray A, Rayner M. The economic burden of coronary heart disease in the U.K. *Heart* 2002; 88:597-603.

64. Thompson D, Wolf AM. The medical-care cost burden of obesity. *Obesity review* 2001; 2:189-197.

65. American Diabetes Association: Direct costs of diabetes (http://www.hhs.gov/news/press/2003pres/20030227 a.html.)

66. Hoffman C, Rice D, Sung H-Y. Persons with chronic conditions: Their prevalence and costs. *JAMA.*1996; 276:1473-1479.

67. *Department of Health: Annual Report 2001/2002,* Pretoria: South Africa Department of Health, 2002.

68. Gumber A and Kulkarni V. *Health Security for Workers: The Case of the Informal Sector.* National Consultation on Health Security in India, July 2001.

69. Pestana JA, Steyn K, Leiman A, Hartzenberg GM. The direct and indirect costs of cardiovascular disease in South Africa in 1991. *S Afr Med J.* 1996; 86:679-684.

70. Jha P, Chaloupka FJ. *Curbing the Epidemic: Governments and the Economics of Tobacco Control.* 1999 The World Bank, Washington, DC

71. Zatonski WA, McMichael AJ, Powles JW. Ecological study of reasons for sharp decline in mortality from ischaemic heart disease in Poland since 1991. *BMJ* 1998;316:1047-1051.

72. Rose G. Sick individuals and sick populations. *Int J Epidemiol.* 1985; 14:32-38

73. Beaglehole R, Yach D. Globalization and the prevention and control of non-communicable disease: the neglected chronic diseases of adults. *Lancet* 2003; 362:903-908.

74. Nissinen A, Berrios X, Puska P. Community-based noncommunicable disease interventions: lessons from developed countries for developing ones. *Bulletin of the WHO* 2001; 79: 963-970.

75. Oster G, Thomspon D. Estimated effects of reducing dietary saturated fat intake on the incidence and costs of coronary heart disease in the U.S. J Am Diet Assoc. 1996;127-131.

76. The WHO. *The World Health Report 2003 Shaping the Future.* Chapter 6: Neglected Global Epidemics: Three Growing Threats. Geneva: the WHO, 2003

77. Puska P. Nutrition and mortality: the Finnish experience. *Acta Cardiol.* 2000; 55:213-220.

78. Ebrahim S and Smith G D Systematic review of randomized controlled trials of multiplerisk factor interventions for preventing coronary heart disease. *BMJ* 1997; 314:1666-1671.

79. Popkin B, Horton S, Kim S. Program options for diet-related interventions to control epidemic, chronic diseases in Asia and the Pacific. *Food and Nutrition Bulletin* 2001; 22 (s): 47-51.

80. Dowse GK Gareeboo H, Alberti KGMM, Zimmett P. et al. Changes in population cholesterol concentrations and other cardiovascular risk factor levels after five years of the non-communicable disease intervention programme in Mauritius. BMJ 1995;311:1255-1259.

81. Kim S, Moon S, Popkin BJ. The nutrition transition in South Korea. *Am J Clin Nutr* 2000;71:44-53.

82. U.K. Prospective Diabetes (UKPDS) Group. Intensive blood-glucose control with sulphonylureas or insulin compared with conventional treatment and risk of complications in patients with type 2 diabetes (UKPDS 33) *Lancet* 1998;352:837-53, and U.K. Prospective Diabetes (UKPDS) Group. Effect of intensive blood glucose control with metformin on complications in overweight patients with type 2 diabetes (UKPDS 34) *Lancet* 1998;352:854-865.

83. Heart Protection Study Collaborative Group. MRC/BHF heart protection study of cholesterol lowering with simvastatin in 20536 high-risk individuals: a randomized placebo-controlled trial. *Lancet* 2002; 360: 7-22.

84. Kostis JB, Davis BR, Cutler J, Grimm RH Jr. et al. Prevention of heart failure by antihypertensive drug treatment in older persons with isolated systolic hypertension. SHEP Cooperative Research Group. *JAMA.* 1997; 278:212-216.

85. Whisnant J.The decline of stroke. *Stroke* 1984;15:160-168.

86. Garg R, Yusef S. Overview of randomized clinical trials of angiotensin-converting enzyme inhibitors in mortality and morbidity in patients with heart failure. *JAMA.* 1995; 273:1450-1456.

87. Shibata MC, Flather MD, Wang D. Systematic review of the impact of beta-blockers on mortality and hospital admissions in heart failure. *Eur J Heart F Ail.* 2001;3:351-357.

88. EUROASPIRE I and II Group. Clinical reality of coronary prevention guidelines: a comparison of EUROASPIRE I and II in nine countries. *Lancet* 2001; 357: 995-1001.

89. Wald NJ, Law MR. A strategy to reduce cardiovascular disease by more than 80%. *BMJ* 2003;326:1419-1424.

90. Neaton JD, Wentworth D. Serum cholesterol, blood pressure, cigarette smoking, and death from coronary heart disease. *Arch Intern Med* 1992;152:56-64.

91. MacMahon S, Peto R, Cutler J, Collins R. et al. Blood pressure, stroke and coronary heart disease, Part I: Effects of prolonged differences in blood pressure - Evidence from nine prospective observational studies corrected for the regression dilution bias. *Lancet* 1990;335:765-774.

92. Lewington S, Clarke R, Qizilbash N, Peto R, Collins R. Prospective Studies Collaboration. Age-specific relevance of usual blood pressure to vascular mortality: a meta-analysis of individual data for one million adults in 61 prospective studies. *Lancet* 2002; 360:1903-1913.

93. Lawes CM, Rodgers A, Bennett DA. et al. Asia Pacific Cohort Studies Collaboration. Blood pressure and cardiovascular disease in the Asia Pacific region. *J Hypertens.* 2003;21:707-716.

94. Collins R, Peto R, MacMahon S, Hebert P. et al. Blood pressure, stroke, and coronary heart disease. Part 2, Short-term reductions in blood pressure: overview of randomised drug trials in their epidemiological context. *Lancet 1990;335(8704):1534-5.*

95. Law MR. Wald NJ. Morris JK. Jordan RE. Value of low does combination treatment with blood pressure lowering drugs: analysis of 354 randomised trials. *BMJ* 2003; 326:1427-1435.

96. Reddy KS. Research for prevention and control of high blood pressure and associated cardiovascular risk factors in the developing countries: summary report of an *IC Health Workshop* October 9-12, 2001, Geneva.

97. LaRosa JC, He J, Vupputuri S, Effect of statins on risk of coronary disease. *JAMA.* 1999; 282:2340-2346.

98. Law MR, Wald NJ, Rudnicka AR. Quantifying effect of statins on low density lipoprotein cholesterol, ischaemic heart disease, and stroke: systematic review and meta-analysis. BMJ 2003;326:1423-1427.

99. Rodgers A. A cure for cardiovascular disease? *BMJ* 2003; 326:1407-1408

100. Greenberg H and Farmer RG. Global Health Assessment: A New Perspective. *Ann Noninvasive Electrocardiol.* 2002;7:73-77.

101. Tuomilehto J, Lindstrom J, Eriksson JG, et al. Prevention of type 2 diabetes mellitus by.changes in lifestyle among subjects with impaired glucose tolerance. *N Engl J Med* 2001;344:1343-1350.

102. Amos AF, McCarty DJ, Zimmet P. The rising global burden of diabetes and its complications: estimates and projections to the year 2010. *Diabet Med.* 1997;14 (suppl5) S1-S85.

103. Ford ES Williamson D Ford ES, Giles WH, Dietz WH. Prevalence of the metabolic syndrome among U.S. adults. *JAMA.* 2002; 287:356-359. and Ford ES, Williamson, DF, Liu S. Weight change and diabetes incidence: findings from a national cohort of U.S. adults *Amer J Epidemiol* 1997;146:214-222

104. Hu FB, Manson JE, Stampfer MJ, Colditz G. et al. Diet, lifestyle, and the risk of type 2 diabetes mellitus in women. *N Engl J Med.* 2001; 345:790-797.

105. Joint editorial ADA, NIHLBI, JDFI et al. Diabetes mellitus: a major risk factor for cardiovascular disease. *Circulation* 1999;100:1132-1133.

106. De Lorgeril M, Salen P, Martin J, Monjaud I. et al. Mediterranean diet, traditional risk factors, and the rate of cardiovascular complications after myocardial infarction. *Circulation* 1999;99:779-785.

107. Singh RB, Rastogi SS, Verma R, et al. Randomised controlled trial of cardioprotective diet in patients with recent acute myocardial infarction. *BMJ.* 1992; 304:1015-1019.

108. Burr ML, Gilbert JF, Holliday RM, et al. Effects of changes in fat, fish, and fiber intakes on death and myocardial infarction: diet and reinfarction trial (DART). *Lancet* 1989;ii:757-761.

109. MW Gillman, LA Cupples, D Gagnon et al. Protective effect of fruits and vegetables on development of stroke in men. *JAMA* 1995 273: 1113-7.

110. Ammerman AS, Lindquist CH, Lohr KN, Hersey J. The efficacy of behavioral interventions to modify dietary fat and fruit and vegetable intake: A review of the evidence. *Prev Med* 2002; 35:25-41.

111. Bowen DJ, Beresford SAA. Dietary intervention to prevent disease. *Ann Rev Public Health* 2002;23:255-286.

112. Halpern MT, Shikiar R, Rentz AM et al. Impact of smoking status on workplace absenteeism and productivity *Tob Control* 2001;10:233- 238.

113. Ezzati M, Lopez AD. Estimates of global mortality attributable to smoking in 2000. *Lancet* 2003; 362: 847-852.

114. Lloyd-Jones DM, Larson MG, Leip EP, et al. Lifetime risk for developing congestive heart failure: The Framingham Heart Study. Circulation 2002; 106:3068-3072.

115. Marshall T. Coronary heart disease prevention: insights from modeling incremental cost-effectiveness. *BMJ* 2003; 327:1264-1267.

116. Covey J and Brown LD. Critical cooperation: an alternative form of civil society-business engagement. *Institute for Development Research Occasional Papers,* 2001;17:1.

117. M Walzer, The Civil Society Argument, *Theorizing Citizenship.* Ed. R Briner. New York; SUNY Press, 1995.

118. Freedom in the World 2003: The annual survey of political rights and civil liberties. (http://www.freedomhouse.org/research)

119. Raymond S. A region in transformation: The political realities of health care management. *J Health Adm Educ.*1994; 12:463-469.

120. Independent Inquiry into Inequalities in Health: Report (Chairman: Sir Donald Acheson) TSO, 1998.